YOUR HEALTH IS YOUR ONLY WEALTH

About the Author

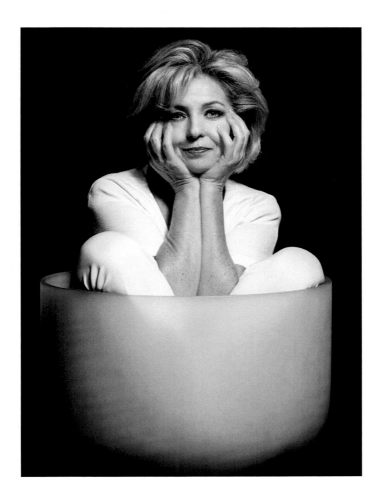

Kimberley Solari is a Reiki Master and Vibrational Sound Healer with over 15 years' experience working with life force energy and quartz crystal singing bowls. She works extensively with cancer patients including paediatrics, with the most incredible results. Her aim is to enlighten the world to the benefits of VSH. Her wish is to be invited to take part in clinical trials.

This book is dedicated to my patients who have trusted me with their health and wellbeing.

Kimberley Solari

YOUR HEALTH IS YOUR ONLY WEALTH

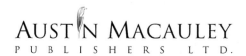

AUSTIN MACAULEY
PUBLISHERS LTD.

Illustrations by Miranda Pothecary
Photographs by Chris Kemp

A CIP catalogue record for this title is available from the British Library.

ISBN 9781785546556 (hardback)
ISBN 9781785546532 (paperback)

www.austinmacauley.com

First Published (2015)

Austin Macauley Publishers Ltd.
25 Canada Square
Canary Wharf
London
E14 5LB

Printed and bound in Great Britain

Contents

Foreword

It was November 2007. I remember thinking my world had just fallen apart. I can recall that phone call like it was yesterday.

My Dad had just telephoned home from the Oxford Radcliffe hospital to tell my mum that he had just been diagnosed with *throat cancer.* All I knew about cancer was that it usually meant someone was going to die; My Dad, surely not! My older brother Tom and my Mum were crying hysterically and they were distraught with grief... as if somebody had already died.

It was in the following week that by fate my Dad met Kimberley (Kimbers to me!). She is a Reiki Master and Vibrational Sound Practitioner, who works with singing quartz crystal healing bowls.

Mum and Dad both immediately immersed themselves in Kimbers' unconditional love and healing. She had an amazing effect on them. Dad was seeing Kimbers on a daily basis for treatment with my Mum, and after returning home after their first session, my parents had both gained so much, including an enormous mental strength which was unbelievable to see after such horrific news, and one that carried them and the rest of our family through my Dad's recovery. Mum and

Dad were acting like his cancer was a walk in the park, which gave the whole entire family such pride and comfort.

At the time of my Dad's diagnosis, I was attending the football academy at Southampton, and I was so worried that my Dad may never see me play professional football as he was my biggest fan! One day after training, Dad's appointment clashed with me getting home, so I joined them in Kimberley's treatment room, and I was blown away by the calmness, peace and energy that I felt, even though I was only 15. I immediately warmed to her, and seven years on the relationship I have with Kimbers is like she's my big sis. Whenever I have a football injury or feel anxious, I always book in to see her, and I'm not slow in coming forward to point my team mates in her direction! And yes, some of my team mates really do go and see her, and they too, have gathered such strength and awareness about her amazing holistic treatment.

As well as Kimbers' treatment, Dad also underwent radiotherapy and chemotherapy. Doctors were constantly amazed by his strength and fortitude (which he put down to Kimbers) and his ability to resist the normal side-effects of his medical treatments.

Kimbers had another string to her bow. She had a psychic ability. This was to amaze us all with her accurate and alluring predictions!

When Dad was first diagnosed he was told that he would have to have a life-saving operation that would leave him disfigured and learning how to eat, speak, and swallow again. Kimbers told him that he would never have this operation (this message came from his mum who was in spirit) and true to form, she was right. The message from his mum told him to seek a second medical opinion. He did this, and to his surprise was informed he could be cured without the need for the horrific operation.

On another occasion, Kimbers had informed Dad that his cancer had gone and that he no longer needed medical treatment. That very evening Dad's oncologist telephoned him to give him the news that following his latest MRI scan, his tumour could no longer be seen and was not present!!

And the story continues... but it's not me writing the book, just the Foreword!

I hope you enjoy reading Kimbers' book as much as I've enjoyed having her in our lives.

James Rowe

Introduction

My name is Kimberley Solari and I am a Vibrational Sound Practitioner, Reiki Master, Mind and Body Tuner and Teacher. I am the architect and visionary behind the Alphasono-Biometrics™ Assessment Programme which is a unique and innovative way of assessing the body's own natural symphony and bringing it back 'on key'.

This book will explain how true health can only be achieved by removing the 'crap' that we've stored in each Chakra from the moment we were born. I use the word 'crap' here, because it really is that! We are unnecessarily hoarding our life's experiences and journeys in our body's energy centres (Chakras).

Reiki is based on channelling life force energy into a living organism, such as the human body. I balance and lift out 'crap' stored within your Chakras and energy field to achieve perfect health. The vibrational tones of the quartz crystal healing bowls allow the continuation of lifting out one's 'crap' once the life force energy has opened up your Chakras. The vibrational tones from the quartz crystal bowls start lifting out and repairing instantaneously on contact with your body's own natural symphony. I have found that working with these two ancient healing methods can really lead to an illness-free life.

As an example, how many of you are walking around wearing your first ever baby-grow? Of course, no one is. However, we are all carrying around in our first Chakra (the root Chakra) the fears and joys we experienced from birth to age seven. Bone and rectal cancers, for example, begin deep within this Chakra. But it truly starts from chronic emotional issues. In this case, this could stem from issues around your parents relationship and the atmosphere they created within the home around you. If it was toxic you would be suffering from personal survival issues and low self-esteem which in adulthood can lead to difficulties in one's ability to settle down in a working environment, or the desire to commit to a long-standing relationship.

Further on in this book there is a clear and concise description of each Chakra and the symptoms you will feel if they are not opened and cleaned out.

It really is important for every reader to understand that by *removing* the clutter that has collected through their life they are helping to ensure that their emotional wellbeing stays 'on key', as well as *ALL* the major organs in the body.

Nobody wants to have **cancer, strokes, heart attacks, diabetes, IBS, ME, MS, or any other disease,** but all the above will occur if we do not take the body's major organ frequencies into account. Are you 'on key' or 'off key'? You are all walking around with your major organs on a knife edge of breaking down due to being 'off key'.

The organ donor list is shrinking, so don't bank on getting one soon if *you* allow your organs to suffer out of neglect and ignorance. I hope this book will revolutionise the way you listen to, think about and treat your body.

The scourge of cancer

There are an estimated 2.5 million people in the UK today (2015) who have had a cancer diagnosis. This is an increase of almost half a million in the previous five years. Worryingly, around one in four (25%) people in the UK already face poor health or disability after treatment for cancer. If this number continues to rise by over 3% a year, this could see four million people living with cancer by 2030.

According to Macmillan Cancer Support more than a thousand people will be diagnosed with cancer *EVERY DAY* in the UK in December 2016 according to a new analysis from Macmillan Cancer Support.

The new figures show that within just two years around 100,000 more people will be diagnosed with cancer each year compared to 20 years ago. In 1996, 263,000 people were diagnosed with cancer and by 2016 this is predicted to grow to a staggering 361,000, equivalent to the entire population of Cardiff being diagnosed each year. The charity warns the NHS will be pushed to its limit by the soaring numbers of cancer patients unless *VITAL ACTION* is taken by the next government.

In the UK an average of around 1,600 children are diagnosed with cancer each year: that's 30 children every week. Around one in 500 children in Great Britain will develop some form of cancer by 14 years of age. Leukaemia is the most commonly diagnosed cancer in children. Leukaemia, brain, other CNS and intracranial tumours and lymphomas account for more than two-thirds of all cancers diagnosed in children. In Great Britain children's cancer incidence rates have increased by more than 40% since the late 1960s. The reasons for this are poorly understood, though improvements in diagnosis and registration are likely to have played a part. Throughout Europe children's cancer incidence rates are lowest in the UK and highest in Northern Europe.

More than one million people in the US get cancer every year (see overleaf).

Each year around 13,500 children are diagnosed with cancer in the US. That's more than a classroom of kids a day. Some 25% of all kids who are diagnosed with cancer die.

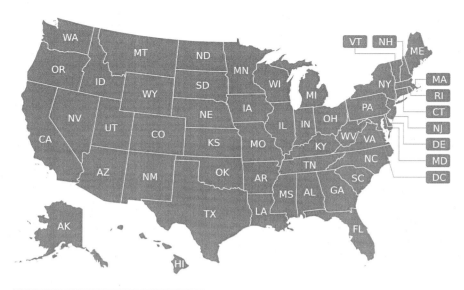

WA 38,180	ID 8,080	MT 5,950	ND 3,840	OK 19,280
MO 34,680	IL 65,460	IN 35,620	WV 11,730	FL 114,040
OR 22,410	NV 13,640	WY 2,860	SD 2,520	TX 113,630
AR 13,830	TN 38,300	KY 26,490	NC 50,420	ME 8,810
CA 172,090	UT 11,050	CO 24,540	NE 9,540	MN 29,730
LA 24,100	MS 16,260	AL 26,150	SC 25,550	NH 8,090
AK 3,070	AZ 32,440	NM 9,970	KS 14,440	IA 17,140
WI 32,700	MI 57,420	OH 65,010	GA 48,070	VT 4,020
NY 107,840	VA 41,170	RI 6,040	NJ 51,410	MD 30,050
HI 6,730	PA 81,540	MA 37,790	CT 21,970	DE 5,280
DC 2,800				

Estimated numbers of new cancer cases from 2015 in the US, excluding basal cell and squamous cell skin cancers and in situ carcinomas except urinary bladder. NOTE: state estimates are offered as a rough guide and should be interpreted with caution. State estimates may not add to US total due to rounding.

Source: www.cancer.org/research/cancerfactactsstatistics/ cancerfactsfigures2015

Disclaimer

Kimberley Solari is *not* a physician and none of the information in this book should be construed as "medical advice". The author is merely presenting her findings, as would an investigative journalist. Thus, the material in this book should be used for educational and informational purposes only. Each person must make his or her own decisions about treatment. Prior to making those decisions, anyone who has or suspects they may have cancer or any other health issues, should consult with a qualified physician.

A conscientious effort has been made to only present information that is accurate and truthful in this book. However, the author cannot be held responsible for inaccuracies that may be found in her source material. Moreover, this is not the only alternative therapy available.

The testimonials in this book (pages 104–37) have been freely given and are a true and honest account of her patients' health changes which have taken place whilst receiving regular treatments under her care and supervision.

The old wives' tale,
'Beauty comes from within',
Is so right.
But wake up people!
So does your health!

Chapter 1

So What on Earth IS Vibrational Medicine?

Vibrational medicine is based on the idea that all illness or disease is characterized by blockages in the channels on some level either in nadis (pronounced *naRdi*), arteries, veins, and nerves. When there is a blockage in the organ in question, the organ's own healthy frequency that it naturally omits is weakened and dulled, and therefore the frequency is slightly lowered, which creates illness and disease.

You can only re-harmonize your own body's healthy frequency by visiting a vibrational sound practitioner, just as you would only have a professional mechanic retune a car's engine. Medication from your GP will not retune a major organ within the body; neither will wrapping a blanket around a car engine that is not functioning properly fix it.

Different frequencies within the body link directly to the colours of our body's aura, and the colours of our Chakras. If a frequency is vibrating fast enough, it's emitted as a colour of light. If we wanted to convert vibrational sound (frequencies) to light, we would simply raise its frequency forty octaves. Most human beings are unable to process these low frequencies and therefore cannot see or recognize another person's aura-field.

Further on in the book these frequencies (the 'notes') and their matching colours will be fully explained.

When two frequencies are brought together, the lower will always rise to meet the higher. This is the principle of resonance. So, when a piano is tuned, a tuning fork is struck, and then brought close to the piano string that carries that same musical tone. The string then raises its vibration automatically and attunes itself to the same rate at which the fork is vibrating (the frequency).

By using clear and frosted quartz crystal healing bowls the above principle of resonance is created and leads to seamless well-being. The tone of a clear set of bowls is that of the ivory (white) notes of the pianos (the true notes), opposed to the frosted bowls which are the black notes on the piano (the sharp notes).

Bringing an unhealthy body back to its true state of wellness happens over time and I do this by using these quartz crystal healing bowls just like the tuning fork with the piano. Your body is the piano, and the healing bowls act like the separate tuning forks that correspond with the frequency (the key on the piano) of your major Chakras. I place a clear bowl on the body, and I surround the body with the frosted bowls. When these bowls are played into the body, the body's major organs naturally recognize the frequency, allowing the organ to retune itself.

When harmonization is occurring with the above frequencies and they are all semi in tune, I will introduce the 528Hz DNA bowl. This will at first create a dissonance where the frequencies are not matching, but I will keep playing until the entire body is in harmony with the 528Hz bowl.

This very important 528Hz healing bowl will be explained further within this book.

Chapter 2

Your Seven Major Chakras

The following pages have been concisely laid out so you can fully understand and appreciate the significance of your Chakras in your well-being and happiness.

ROOT CHAKRA

The vibrational note of this Chakra is C and C#.
It resonates to the frequency of the colour **red**, and it will appear this colour on a Chakra photograph.

The base, or root, Chakra is located between the anus and the genitals. For a female, the root Chakra governs the ovaries. For a male, it governs the genitals. This Chakra begins to bud the moment we are born into this world and absorbs everything we feel, hear and smell, right up to the age of seven. At the age of seven, it is completely full.

On an emotional level, this Chakra becomes congested with thoughts and stress concerning survival, tribal issues, and instinct, past life issues, family, marriage, parenting, correct behaviour, society and the ability to provide basic needs for living.

As a person begins to grow up, perhaps finding themselves in a relationship or engaging in family/ friend relationships, the stress of following the establishment and the family's rules, or doing what their family/spouse wants, becomes too much. The pressure of trying to fit in at home, school, work etc., compounded by any compromises to the above, will put huge pressure on the root Chakra. Subsequently, the physical areas of the body governed by this Chakra can become at risk.

When the Root Chakra is congested with the above fears, it can develop into a person suffering from minor, or major, health problems in the body pertaining to blood, bone or immune disorders. Issues also include cancers in the rectal area, the vagina (cervical cancer), genitals (testicular cancer), chronic pain in the base of the spine, sciatica (lower back pain), feet and leg problems (varicose veins, leg cramps), and emotional issues including depression. Issues with infertility also arise when this Chakra becomes unhealthy.

It can become an almost perpetual cycle, where emotional issues have led to physical issues, but these physical issues may lead to more emotional issues – you may find yourself in a tumultuous 'Catch 22' if you don't address the needs of this Chakra!

If the Root Chakra is closed, it will appear black on an imaging photograph. For females, they could experience fertility issues, digestive problems, and for males, they could experience fertility issues, urinary tract infections and prostate cancer.

If you have mild, or major, symptoms of any of the above, then your **Root** Chakra needs to be emptied. This can be done by visiting a Reiki Master/Practitioner, or a Vibrational Sound Practitioner.

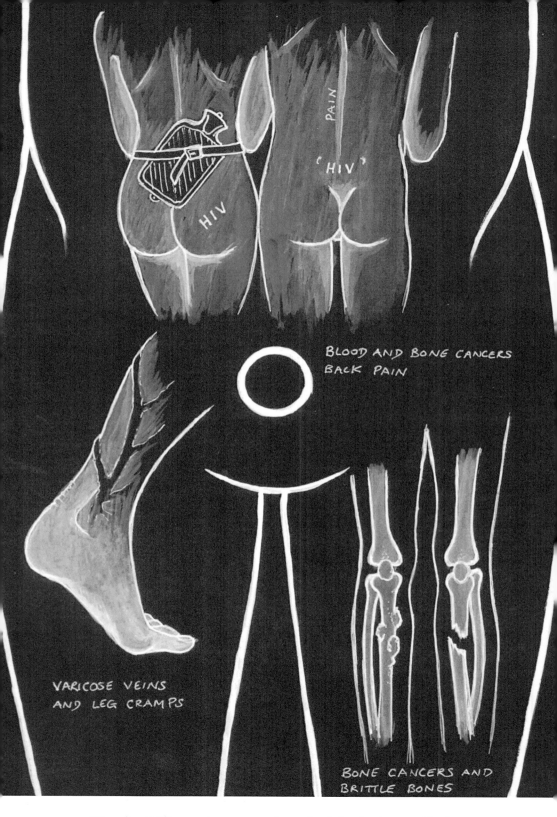

Physical Ailments – associated with the Root Chakra

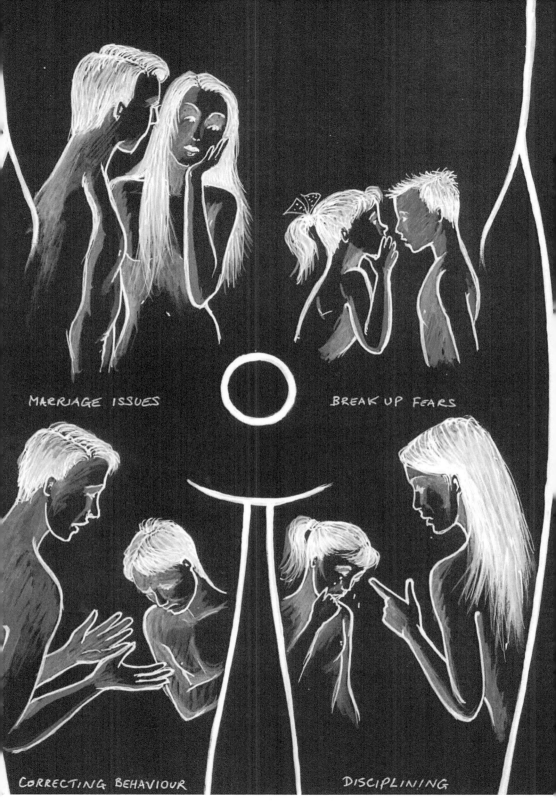

Emotional Issues – associated with the Root Chakra

SACRAL CHAKRA

The vibrational note of this Chakra is D and D#.
It resonates to the frequency of the colour **burnt orange**, and it will appear this colour on a Chakra photograph.

The Sacral Chakra is located between the belly button and the genitals. It governs the bladder, small intestines, large intestines and kidneys. This Chakra activates just after the age of seven and is full by the time we reach our teens.

On an emotional level, this Chakra becomes congested with thoughts and stress concerning power, creativity, sexual issues, blame, control, passion, ethics, money, greed, honour in relationships, fidelity, feelings of repression or wrongness in sexual matters and birthing new ideas.

As one begins to explore the freedom our parents entrust in us, we are empowered, or 'egged on', by our peers to discover things that are beyond our years and understanding. The pressure to comply or rebel against some of the above elements can become overwhelming – not only in our younger years, but also as an adult. This puts strain on the Sacral Chakra.

When stress relating to the above factors becomes too much, the physical areas of the body governed by this Chakra can become affected. Problems can include impacts to the reproductive organs, cancers in this area, erectile issues, pelvic and lower back pains, urinary and bladder problems and issues with the hips.

If the Sacral Chakra is closed, it will appear black on an imaging photograph. You may experience issues with the desire to eat, going to the bathroom properly and power issues within your work and personal life.

If you have mild, or major, symptoms of any of the above, then your **Sacral** Chakra needs to be cleared. This can be done by visiting a Reiki Master/Practitioner, or a Vibrational Sound Practitioner.

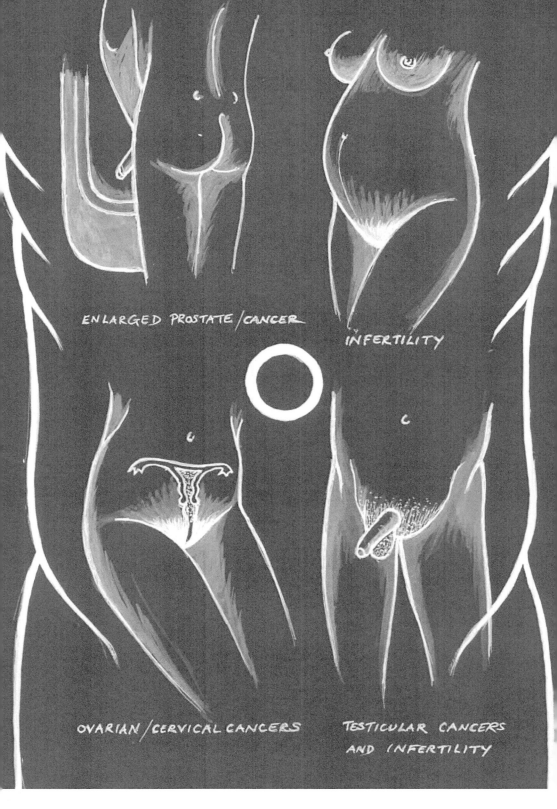

Physical Ailments – associated with the Sacral Chakra

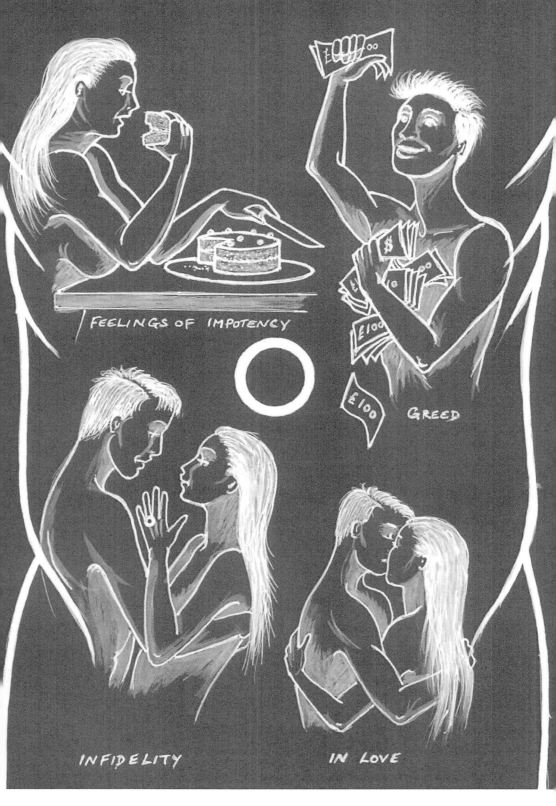

Emotional Issues – associated with the Sacral Chakra

SOLAR PLEXUS CHAKRA

The vibrational note of this Chakra is E and E#.
It resonates to the frequency of the colour yellow, and
it will appear this colour on a Chakra photograph.

The Solar Plexus Chakra is located above the belly
button, above the Sacral Chakra. It governs the
stomach, the spleen and the liver. This Chakra is
activated from around the age we start communicating,
approximately three years old, and remains so until we
die.

On an emotional level, this Chakra deals with
responsibility issues, caring for others, trust, fear,
guilt, career, intimidation, personal honour, feelings
of victimization and courage. It also pertains to self-
concern issues, self-respect, sensitivity to criticism,
self-esteem, self-worth and our confidence.

Stress, **strain** and **hassle** are the main catalysts for
ailments in this area.

Physical issues related to this Chakra include
indigestion, stomach problems, intestinal and colon
problems, eating disorders, diabetes, arthritis, adrenal
issues, dysfunctions with the liver and pancreas,
issues with the gall bladder, kidneys and ulcers. It can
also include dysfunctions in the spleen and mid-back
problems.

Our spleen is a very important organ as it regulates the healthy composition of your blood, which plays an important role in carrying oxygen around your body and brain, helps in blood clotting, and also aids the immune system, so problems with this Chakra will lead to problems resulting from unhealthy blood flow, such as leukaemia, cysts, rheumatoid arthritis and other problems.

When this Chakra is closed, it will appear black on an imaging photograph. One may experience depression through responsibility issues, or feeling burdened by such issues.

If you have mild, or major, symptoms of any of the above, then your Solar Plexus Chakra needs to be cleared. This can be done by visiting a Reiki Master/ Practitioner, or a Vibrational Sound Practitioner.

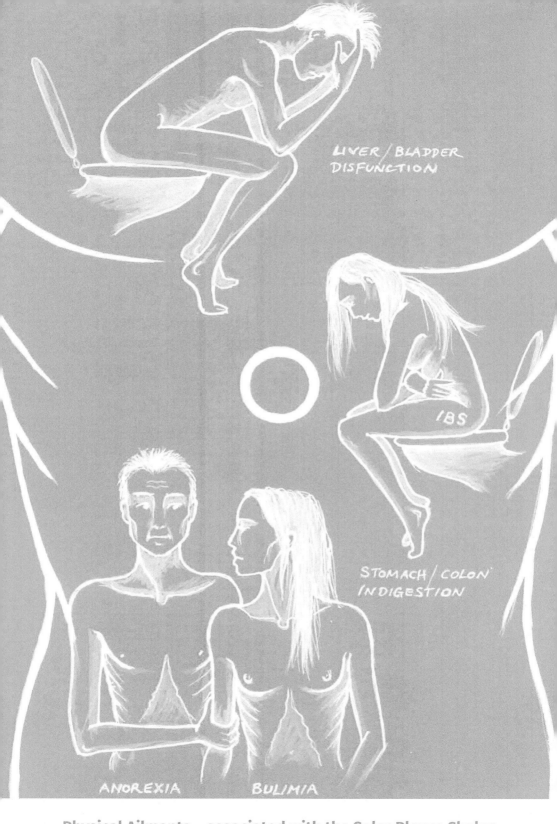

Physical Ailments – associated with the Solar Plexus Chakra

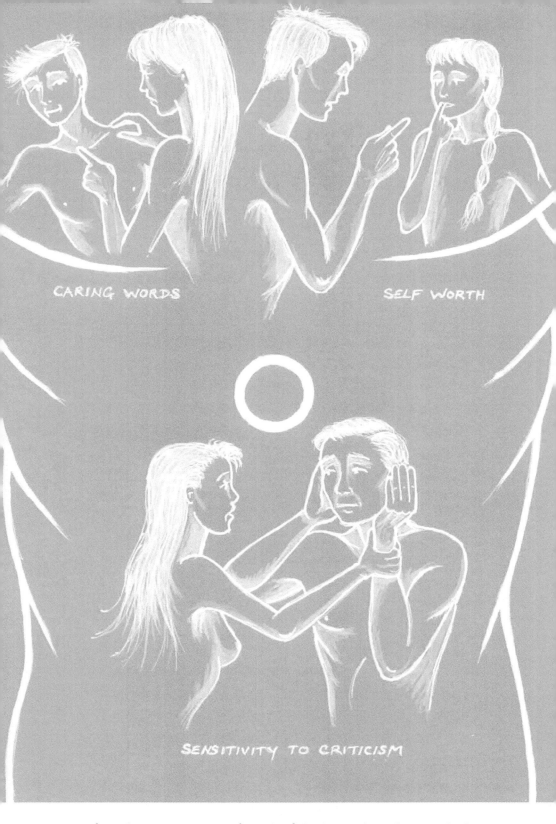

CARING WORDS

SELF WORTH

SENSITIVITY TO CRITICISM

Emotional Issues – associated with the Solar Plexus Chakra

HEART CHAKRA

The vibrational note of this Chakra is F and F#.
It resonates to the frequency of the colour green, and it
will appear this colour on a Chakra photograph.

The Heart Chakra is located between the lower parts
of your lungs, nestled just beneath the bottom of your
ribcage. This Chakra is active from birth to death.

On an emotional level, it deals with love, happiness,
desire for happiness, sadness, anger, hatred, prejudice,
loneliness, forgiveness, compassion, hope, desires,
wants, grief, resentment, commitment, trust in your
close interpersonal relationships and your choices in
love.

The emotional issue of prejudice is often instilled into
us at a young age by our parents. This is mainly due to
the way our parents try to bestow their beliefs upon
us, which were conditioned into them by *their* parents.
The rest of the emotional issues are fears that are
transmitted into us through the umbilical cord via our
mothers...

Physical issues related to this Chakra include problems
with the heart and circulatory system, the lungs and
breathing problems, the chest area, breasts, asthma
and associated allergies, pneumonia, bronchitis, upper
back, shoulder and arm problems.

When this Chakra is closed, it appears black on an imaging photograph. Chronic issues when this Chakra is closed include angina, breathing problems, a fear to interact with loved ones and a sense of feeling alone.

If you have mild, or major, symptoms of any of the above, then your Heart Chakra needs to be cleared. This can be done by visiting a Reiki Master/Practitioner, or a Vibrational Sound Practitioner.

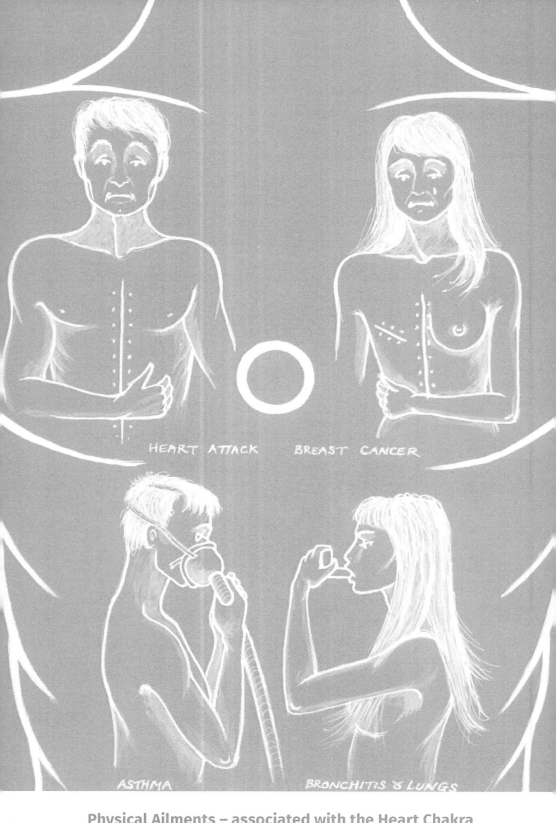

HEART ATTACK   BREAST CANCER

ASTHMA   BRONCHITIS & LUNGS

Physical Ailments – associated with the Heart Chakra

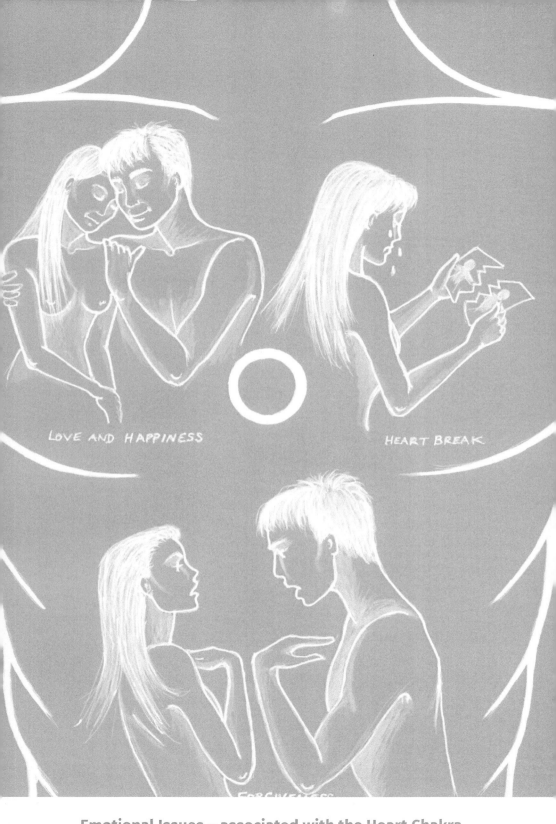

Emotional Issues – associated with the Heart Chakra

THROAT CHAKRA

The vibrational note of this Chakra is G and G#.
It resonates to the frequency of the colour blue, and it
will appear this colour on a Chakra photograph.

The Throat Chakra is located where the Adam's apple is
traditionally found. Like the Heart Chakra, this Chakra is
active from birth to death.

On an emotional level, this Chakra may harbour issues
relating to communication, expressing yourself, telling
the truth to self and others, following your dreams
and being true to yourself. It also relates to addictions,
habits, judgement, faith, making decisions, knowing
and being yourself, criticism, will power, doing what
you say you will do and all forms of expression and
communication.

On a physical level, issues can include problems in
the neck area, mouth, teeth and gums. Thyroid and
gland problems are associated with this Chakra, as are
general issues with the throat, the oesophagus, hiatal
hernias, choking, gagging, sore throats, laryngitis and
all throat and mouth cancers.

When the Throat Chakra starts closing through the
inability of the human being to express their true
selves and feelings, a **hiatal hernia** can occur. This
health issue demonstrates how the Chakras interact

on a vibrational level. The will, or desire, to speak any truth comes from the energy of the solar plexus interacting with the Heart and the Throat Chakras.

This Chakra also appears black on an imaging photograph when closed. One may experience excessive weight gain, bleeding gums and loosening teeth, halitosis and ear infections.

If you have mild, or major, symptoms of any of the above, then your Throat Chakra needs to be cleared. This can be done by visiting a Reiki Master/Practitioner, or a Vibrational Sound Practitioner.

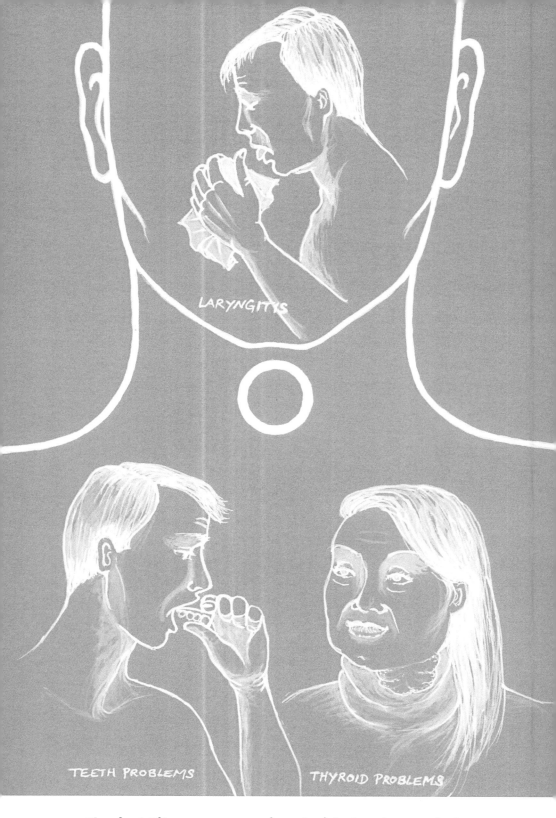

LARYNGITIS

TEETH PROBLEMS

THYROID PROBLEMS

Physical Ailments – associated with the Throat Chakra

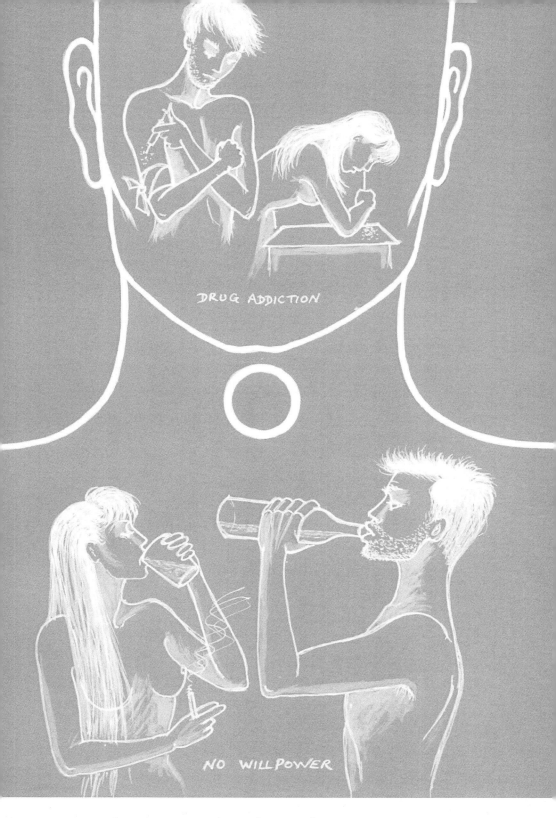

Emotional Issues – associated with the Throat Chakra

THIRD EYE CHAKRA

The vibrational note of this Chakra is A and A#.
It resonates to the frequency of the colour **indigo**, and
it will appear this colour on a Chakra photograph.

The Third Eye Chakra is located in the middle of the
brow. This Chakra becomes active from approximately
the age of three, right through to death.

On an emotional level, this Chakra pertains to issues
with truth, knowledge, intellect, intuitive powers,
learning from experience, feeling inadequate, inner
wisdom, knowing oneself and self-evaluation. It deals
with open-mindedness, accepting yourself and others,
and listening and seeing openly.

On a physical level, issues may include the ears,
hearing problems and mild or even severe tinnitus. Eye
problems can occur, including sensitivity to light and
issues with sight. The nose, brain and nervous system
can also be affected, as can the entire length of the
spine and one's ability to learn.

Again, this Chakra will appear black on an imaging
photograph if closed. Issues may include chronic
migraines, blurred vision and an inclination to withdraw
from people. Additionally, the issue may be an inability
to see and embrace your future.

If you have mild, or major, symptoms of any of the above, then your **Third Eye** Chakra needs to be cleared. This can be done by visiting a Reiki Master/Practitioner, or a Vibrational Sound Practitioner.

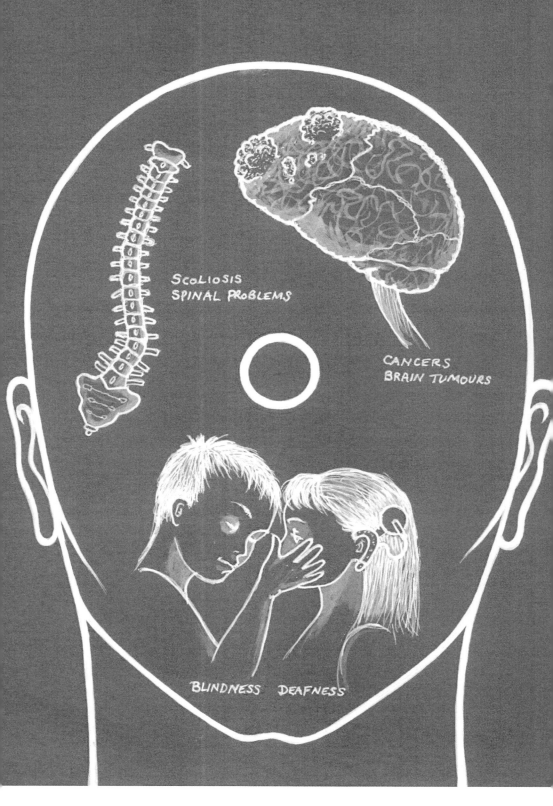

Physical Ailments – associated with the Third Eye Chakra

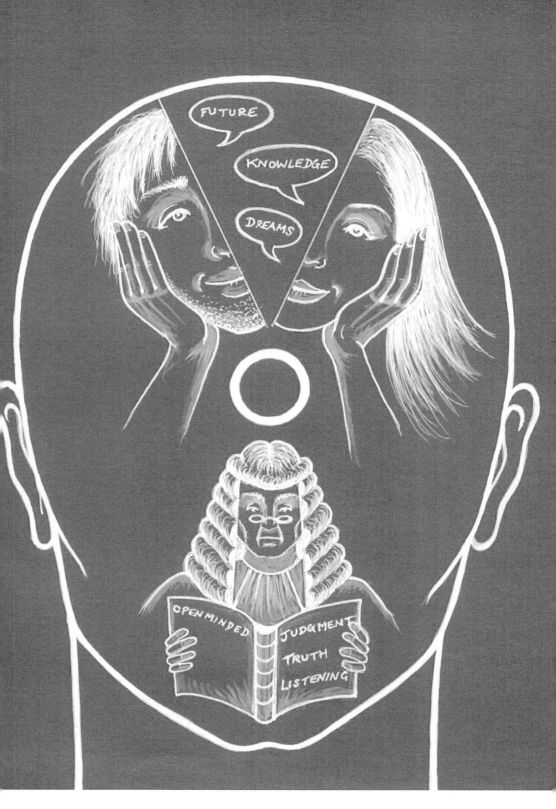

Emotional Issues – associated with the Third Eye Chakra

CROWN CHAKRA

The vibrational note of this Chakra is B and B#.
It resonates to the frequency of the colour white, and it
will appear this colour on a Chakra photograph.

This Chakra is located on the crown of your head. It is
active from birth to death.

On an emotional level, issues with this Chakra can
include spirituality and devotion to personal matters,
unconditional love to self, to others and to nature.
It includes empathy, humanitarianism, selflessness,
values and ethics.

This Chakra also pertains to one's connection with
universal love, energy and knowledge, one's ability to
go with the flow of life and to see the larger picture, our
inspirations without wants and the Higher Self.

On a physical level, problems can include effects to
the body tissue and muscle system, energy/fatigue
and exhaustion problems, mystical depression and
'searching' feelings, sensitivity to the sun, light and
sound.

This Chakra will appear black on an imaging
photograph when closed. Issues from a closed Crown
Chakra include experiencing 'haziness', sleepwalking

through life, being detached from your true self and a fear of embracing your journey on this Earth plane.

If you have mild, or major, symptoms of any of the above, then your Crown Chakra needs to be cleared. This can be done by visiting a Reiki Master/Practitioner, or a Vibrational Sound Practitioner.

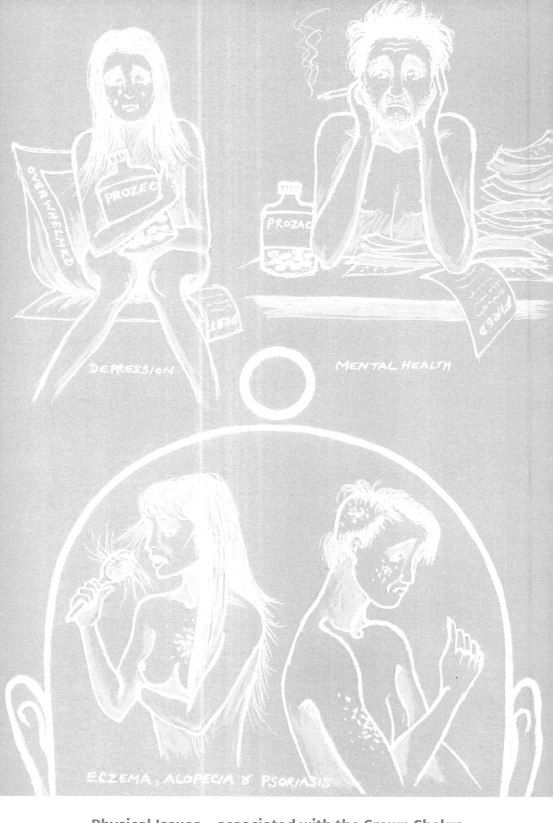

Physical Issues – associated with the Crown Chakra

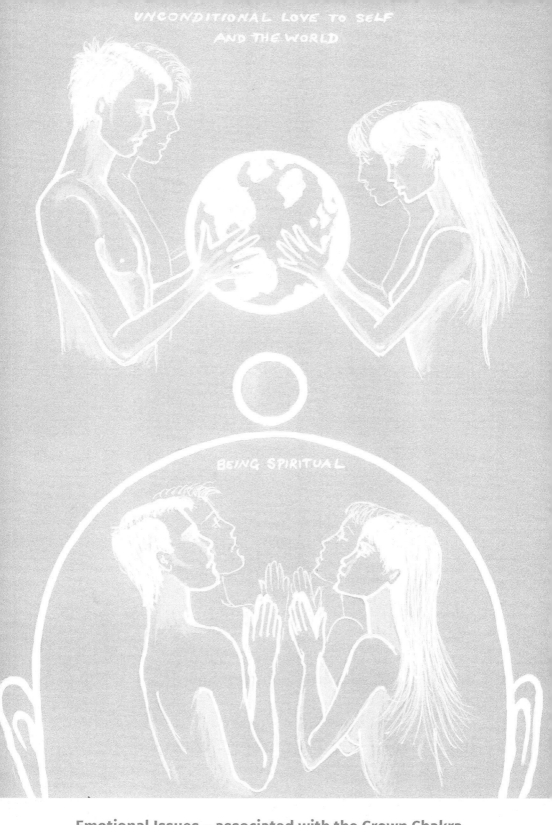

Emotional Issues – associated with the Crown Chakra

Chapter 3

Vibrational Sound Healing

Quartz Crystal Bowl's vibrational frequencies are a form of sound therapy, based on the principle that all matter which has an atomic structure, such as the human body, is in a state of vibration, and the frequency at which an organ or a person most naturally vibrates is called its *resonance*.

The Chakras, bones and organs in the body ALL possess a different resonance frequency and tone.

When an organ is vibrating out of sync or balance, disease is created. The body is in a healthy state of being when each cell and each organ creates a resonance that is in harmony with the whole body. Sound and vibrational treatment is an option that has been proven to have an amazing effect on patients and is considered a safe and complementary treatment to all conventional and holistic therapy.

By creating vibrational sounds, we can directly control fluids such as blood and lymph, influence both the endocrine system (the control and production of hormones), the metabolism AND even manipulate tissues in the human body.

This technology blends the worlds of vibrational medicine with today's "hard core science" to bring about significant ways of healing the body. In the pages following I will explain how these amazing frequencies **DO** and **CAN** heal your body of everything from cancer to the body's natural ageing process, and everything in between. Ignoring this beautiful and gentle healing method is the biggest form of ignorance in the 21st century.

You first need to understand how the vibrational frequencies of the quartz crystal healing bowls relate to the Chakras and therefore every major part of your body.

The Solfeggio scale is used in the making of the quartz crystal healing bowls. This scale, covered in the next chapter, will help you navigate through this part of the book.

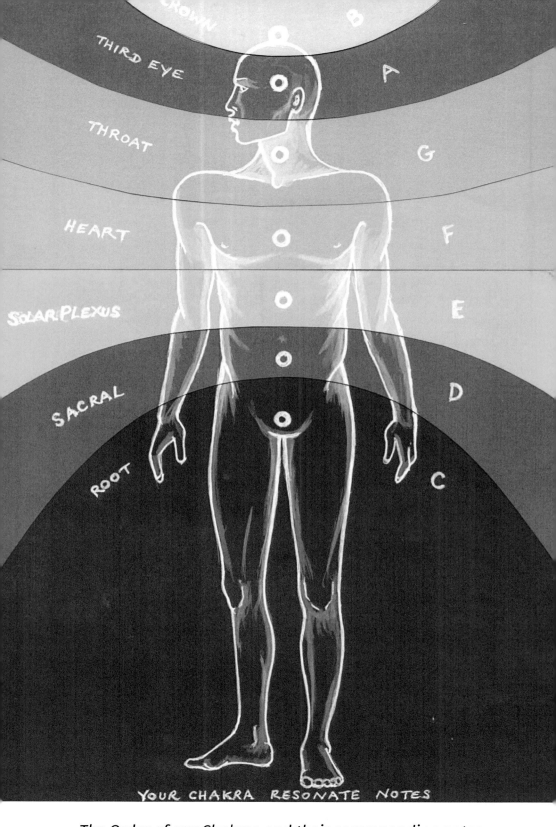

The Order of our Chakras and their corresponding notes

Chapter 4

The Solfeggio Scale

The Solfeggio scale was invented to discover the pitch of a note or true note. It is made of seven different frequencies that are different from the ones in the modern scales that we know of today; do-re-mi-fa-sol-la-ti, which in English translate as C-D-E-F-G-A-B.

The true notes are included in the table on the following page, but please be aware that the quartz crystal healing bowls will naturally resonate within a range of a semitone higher and lower of the true note, while being played on and around the body. This is also a quick guide to the main qualities that match your Chakras. Parts of the text for the great "Hymn to St John the Baptist", from which the names used in the Solfeggio scale are derived, are also given in the table. This chant and its special tones were believed to impart special spiritual blessing when sung in harmony during religious mass. These seven frequencies of the Solfeggio scale can be heard in this hymn, which is why it is believed to have healing and calming properties.

(The colours of the Solar Plexus and the Heart Chakras overlap between yellowish and greenish colours.)

Lyrics	Note Name	Frequency (Hz)	Piano Note	Chakra	Quality
Sancte Iōhannēs	Ti	963	B	Crown	Spirituality
Labiī reātum	La	852	A	Third Eye	Intuition
Solve pollūtī	Sol	741	G	Throat	Truth
Famulī tuōrum	Fa	639	F	Heart	Love
Mīra gestōrum	Mi	528	E	Solar Plexus	Communication
Resonāre fibrīs	Re	417	D	Sacral	Responsibility
Ut queant laxīs	Ut	396	C	Root	Survival

48

An example of a chant from "The Hymn of St John the Baptist" can be listened to by scanning the QR code below.

The frequency 528Hz relates to the note Mi in the scale and comes from the phrase "Mi-ra gestorum", in Latin meaning **miracle**. Stunningly, this is the exact miracle frequency used by genetic biochemists to repair damaged DNA – the genetic blueprint upon which life is based.

The passage below is taken from Dr Leonard Horowitz's book *The Book of 528: Prosperity Key of LOVE*:

"The Western medical paradigm is terminally ill," says Horowitz, "and it's time for a 'miracle' to take its place." That miracle happens to be the "MI" frequency of the ancient Solfeggio musical scale–528Hz frequency, he argues:

"The planet has been poisoned by spiritually-deprived psychopaths lusting for power, profits, and the most effective methods to covertly control populations through petrochemical-pharmaceutical intoxications, and distressing musical vibrations, endangering everything," he asserts.

The alternative, according to Horowitz's text and his *Natural Cure for Global Warming*, is readily doable and deserved by loving intelligent people worldwide. It comes with the understanding that LOVE'S – "The Universal Healer" – is energy (frequency) of sound and light, activating DNA and sustaining biology. That is "528" to be exact, felt in people's hearts and played by increasing numbers of musicians worldwide.

Lennon and LOVE/528 Power

It was recently determined by a fellow 528 researcher and music therapist, who goes under the name "Lunartunar," that John Lennon recorded his famous song, "Imagine", in 528Hz frequency.

This finding means that Lennon learned about this sound of LOVE/528Hz; the sound that Horowitz calls "God's 'C' Note"; the 528Hz "Mi" tone reputed to produce MIRACLES by definition in Solfeggio musicology.

Horowitz speculates that Lennon's "Imagine", along with his "Working Class Hero" campaign, was too much for the war-makers to tolerate, so they had him killed.

The doctor proposes that "'Imagine' energizes the heart in C=528Hz," and produces miraculous manifestations of what is faithfully imagined, envisioned, and intended, especially when administered musically in groups, or even broadcast through the media. Since 528 resonates at the heart of everything, Dr Horowitz reasons, it must be "pure tone LOVE" – "the acoustic channel that links human hearts to the centre of creation, that is God's heart, empowering loving intention to be expressed most powerfully by faithful prayer; commonly observed to manifest miracles." LOVE/528Hz resonates, for example, at the heart of the sun that was recorded by NASA scientists. This can be discerned by comparing the NASA recording with a 528 tuning fork and healing bowl.

Incredibly, according to Horowitz's theories and discoveries, light and sound are synchronized universally at 528 frequencies. 528Hz, he proposes, may be the "zero point" energy that challenges astrophysicists with discoveries of "black holes." Without 528Hz, there would be no circles, nor ability to measure space/time. 528Hz frequency plays a key role in generating the mathematical constants pi (π), phi (φ) and the Fibonacci series, and appears to solve the mystery of the "Pythagorean Comma" – the reason the

Gregorian calendar is imperfect, requiring a "leap year" to adjust the time schedule.

528Hz is the reason there are precisely *5280* feet in a mile, and snowflakes crystallize as six-pointed stars.

In fact, the colour green-yellow is associated with the Solar Plexus and Heart Chakra, and the frequency 528. Dr Horowitz explains. "That is why chlorophyll, which is green-yellow, is the most powerful healing pigment in biology. This is why people and animals eat plants and grass to regain health, and why the air you breathe (oxygen from plants) is the "'prana" of life', or the 'chi' in oriental medicine, like Reiki, and it is filled with the holy aloha spirit of LOVE, vibrating in 528, sending spiritual signals for sustenance through your blood, restoring and invigorating every strand of DNA and cell in your body."

How does Vibrational Sound actually work?

People who can see or feel Life Force energy will tell you that it moves through us in ways that do not always directly relate to the physical structure of our bodies.

We can feel all of the biological processes going on in our body. This includes energy from our food being carried through the blood and being exchanged in chemical processes in all of our body's cells, and also tiny electrical currents of impulses flowing through the brain and being carried along our nerves to move our body and cause it to react to our life and emotions.

Unfortunately most of us cannot physically see the subtler more important energies that are called Life Force energies unless you have been attuned to Reiki and taught by a Reiki Master who feels and sees these energies.

These circulating flows of Life Force energy move in very specific routes around our body, and they feed our organs and tissues. These specific routes are called the Chakras.

Around the physical body there are also layers of multi-coloured light that comprise the Human aura and they are linked with the Chakras and their colours. There are dark clouds of disturbances in these Chakras and auras that are the beginnings of physical illness before they manifest into what we see as physical matter. These dark clouds are blockages that have manifested over time and are preventing the free flow of Life Force energy through your body.

If Life Force energy cannot flow through your body, disease, depression and other serious conditions are created as a survival mechanism – not a curse.

As a Vibrational Sound Practitioner and a Reiki Master, I can read these Life Force energies in the body, and translate them into a language that is easily understood by my patients.

The quartz crystal healing bowls also speak a language of resonance which I can interpret into basic words of understanding for my patients, about how their major organs are functioning.

My bowls sit proudly in silence until they are played. Once played, they become an amazing force of detection. There is nowhere to hide once their vibrational tone starts singing – or *talking*. That's right, I truly do mean talking. Whenever one or more than one bowl is being played, they truly are talking to each other about what's going on deep within you. My keen ear is able to interpret their conversations, and then I can repeat them back to the patient.

By listening to the resonance of the waves of a singing bowl after it has travelled through the body, I can determine the mass of a cancer tumour and its state of reduction by listening intently to the depth of how long the true note is carried through that particular organ affected in the body. I can also determine the health of all the major organs this way, whether the organs are cancerous or not.

Cancer tumours after vibrational sound treatment will become coated with a layer of crystal like substance, which will encase the tumour and prevent the spread of the disease. Cancer needs room to spread, and when it is prevented in doing so, by this encapsulation, the cancer cells then die off. This modification will, on a standard black and white scan image, show that the tumour has enlarged slightly. Oncologists need to increase their awareness of innovative alternative treatments like quartz crystal vibrational sound healing, and the effect that they have on live cancer cells. The one thing neither of us wants to happen is that a patient is given overdoses of chemotherapy, just because their oncologists are uneducated in the world of vibrational sound.

Each time a patient is treated with vibrational sound healing, using quartz crystal healing bowls, the crystallizing resonance enters the body and vibrates through our skin, organs and blood stream, and then attaches itself to the foreign matter, encapsulating it in a layer of crystallization. Chemotherapy acts like boiling water when given to a patient who has a crystallized tumour. The crystalline substance "melts" with the dead cancer cells, and therefore the patient is in remission, and cancer-free. This phenomenon will be highlighted in one of the testimonials at the end of this book.

Chapter 5

Your Unique Symphony

Are you aware that you have a unique symphony?

What do I mean by 'Symphony' and how does it relate to you as a human being? And how would you know if your symphony was 'on key' or 'off key'?

Well, let me explain.

We are born with our own pure and gentle symphony; however our parents' and siblings' symphonies will be mature and 'off key'. As you rush to greet and welcome the new addition into the family, be mindful of how your 'off key' symphony will react with the pure and gentle symphony of the newborn. The baby's symphony will be out of sync with the rest of the family until the baby has adjusted to the layers of symphony echoing around them. Until the new born has adjusted, the baby may show symptoms of excessive crying, irregular sleep patterns, a refusal to take milk and colic. The reason this happens is because the baby is unable to absorb the 'off key' symphonies surrounding them at any one time. The way to avoid this tsunami disaster of trauma, both for yourself and the newborn, is to have your body re-attuned, just like a piano, so that you are 'on key'. An 'on key' family will be very happy, loving, and healthy.

'On key' means your body's symphony is in perfect harmony so your mind can embrace all possibilities and you are a very optimistic person that will say yes to everything to fulfil your zest for life. Being in perfect harmony means you are in excellent health and fulfilling your full potential as an individual.

'Off key' means your body is struggling with health issues; you are in a state of mind where you feel unfulfilled and alone, and have addictions such as binge eating, drinking and taking prescription drugs and narcotics.

If you feel your body is 'off key' then please explore the possibility that you may need to seek the help of somebody like myself, who is an expert in re-tuning your 'off key' symphony.

Your chord and scale relates directly to your health, career and relationship choices.

As you read through my book you will see that the chapters on the human Chakra system have been introduced to you with the corresponding vibrational/

musical note, for example G and G# for the throat Chakra.

The next time you open your mouth to talk try and listen to the octave of your throat note which is G. Is the octave of your voice coming out flat, sharp or soft? Understanding the pitch and tone of your voice will help you to understand the concept of your 'Symphony'.

Do not forget, when you meet somebody for the first time they will take away two impressions of you. The first is your appearance and the second is the pitch and tone of your voice. Is it friendly, is it aggressive, or is it meek and timid? Thinking back on it, have you ever missed out on your dream job for no obvious reason? Have you been unsuccessful in sustaining a meaningful relationship, again for no apparent reason? Could it be the pitch and tone of your voice? Have you found yourself turning off the radio or television because the presenter's voice is grating on you? Are you becoming disengaged and distracted at work? Could it be the pitch and tone of their voices causing these reactions? If yes, it just goes to show that the pitch and tone of our voices have major consequences for what we will and won't tolerate over time.

Next time you have friends over, why not play a game of 'pitch & tone' and see which one appears to you to be friendly, aggressive, meek or timid. This can be done by sitting around a table with your eyes shut and just allowing your ears and heart to listen to the pitch and tone of the person speaking. You can mark each voice by how it made you feel and see if the one you felt was the harshest, the friendliest, the most sympathetic, and the most loving is matched with the rest of the people around the table. Should you find that a certain person's voice has been marked by the majority as sounding aggressive, you can always, with their permission, drill down into that person's experiences to see what has shaped that pitch and tone.

Remember, the 'pitch' and 'tone' of your symphony can be re attuned by coming to see a Vibrational Sound Master practitioner, like myself. My AlphaSono Biometrics Assessment Programme™ has been devised to help you to pinpoint where, in your symphony, you are resonating 'off key' and the reasons why.

A person does not hear sound only through his ears. He hears sound through every pore of his body. It permeates the entire being and according to its particular influence either slows or quickens the rhythm of the blood circulation; it either weakens or soothes the nervous system. It arouses a person to greater passions or it calms him by bringing him peace. According to the sound and its influence a certain effect is produced. Sound becomes visible in the form of radiance. This shows that the same energy which goes into the form of sound before being visible is absorbed by the physical body. In that way the physical body replicates and becomes charged with new magnetism.
Hazrat Inayat Khan (*Mysticism of Sound*)

Your personal chord and scale

You can find your own personal chord and scale by writing out your full birth name and using the letters to find the notes within your name.

For those of you who are not musically minded, a *chord* is a harmonic set of three or more notes that are heard as if sounding simultaneously. A *scale* is a series of notes differing in pitch according to a specific pattern (in this case, the arrangement and pattern of letters in your name) one after the other in a rising or descending order.

For example: Kim**be**rley **Elle**n M**a**tth**e**ws:

Chord = B E A

Scale = B E E E E A E

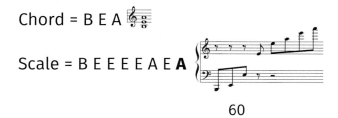

Once married, your new last name is added on the end, and added to the end of your scale and to your chord. For example:

Kim**be**rley **Elle**n M**a**tth**e**ws Sol**a**ri:

Chord = B E A

Scale = B E E E E A E **A**

You can work out your main personal qualities by looking at the notes in the Solfeggio scale on page 48, and the quick references to your personal qualities.

I have one B and two As, which represent intuition and spirituality, and my 5 Es are an indication that I am a confident communicator, spiritually, socially, personally and professionally. These qualities also make me an inspiring and engaging teacher.

Chapter 6

Sports Injuries and Other Major Traumas to the Body

Anyone who plays sport for a living or just for fun, experiences frustration and depression when they are side lined through injury. I treat a lot of young professional footballers and the one thing they all have in common, despite the severity of their injury, is: "When can I get back on the pitch, Kimbers?"

Being picked for the first team of any sport is a privilege for a player, and they hold and take that responsibility with honour and respect. However, the fight to keep their spot in the first team is extremely stressful to a player because they know they have a team mate who is on the bench or sitting in the bleachers waiting for their opportunity to shine. This mental pressure can take a toll both physically and mentally and that is why the players that I see recommend my treatment to their team mates.

My treatment expedites the healing process whilst also working on their emotional and mental state. Once a player is injured they could be looking at months of being side lined but that time frame is shortened by my bespoke healing model. How does this happen?

It happens because my healing treatment repairs the body's DNA. When the body receives trauma injuries our DNA tries to work overtime to repair the damage. This can be a slow and laborious process but by using a 528hz vibrational healing bowl, the process of healing is expedited and the time side lined is reduced, which not only helps the player to regain their position within the team and to help them reach their goals, but it also strengthens their physical and mental state.

Repairing the Body's DNA

DNA, or deoxyribonucleic acid, is the genetic material in humans and almost all other organisms. It is basis of creating all cells in our body.

Cells that are cancerous and mutilated by the onslaught of toxins in our environment, and that have negative emotional baggage, have an extremely damaging effect on our bodies. Many people have compared human DNA to the internet. It communicates immense amounts of information in very small, but significant ways, mimicking a vast network of information portals, not unlike the billions of websites connected to one another all over the world. It may account for our intuition, spontaneous healing, and a number of other phenomena that mainstream science is just beginning to understand. While certainly an interesting idea to think about, hard evidence that frequency and vibrational sound can directly affect DNA and the body's healing processes is still imminent, and as you continue reading this book, my own case studies will add this evidence.

Vibrational sound is not an easy theory to prove or disprove scientifically, and the answers are unlikely to satisfy everyone. The best that we can see is that truth is relative to personal experience in some ways, and when an individual has spiritual and cosmic experiences that do not fall within the explainable territory of rigid science, they are unfortunately ignored by a world that is adamant on disproving fact.

This is a complicated and sometimes heated topic where holistic medicine is constantly being undermined by scientists, consultants and GPs to increase the sales of prescription drugs, and therefore increase the brain's dependency on drug-induced quick fixes that never get to the root of the problem.

At the same time, the human race is coming up against conflicted opinions in how to understand the body at a spiritual level, which means we must be willing to explore the validity of the information received from vibrational sound and spiritual experiences.

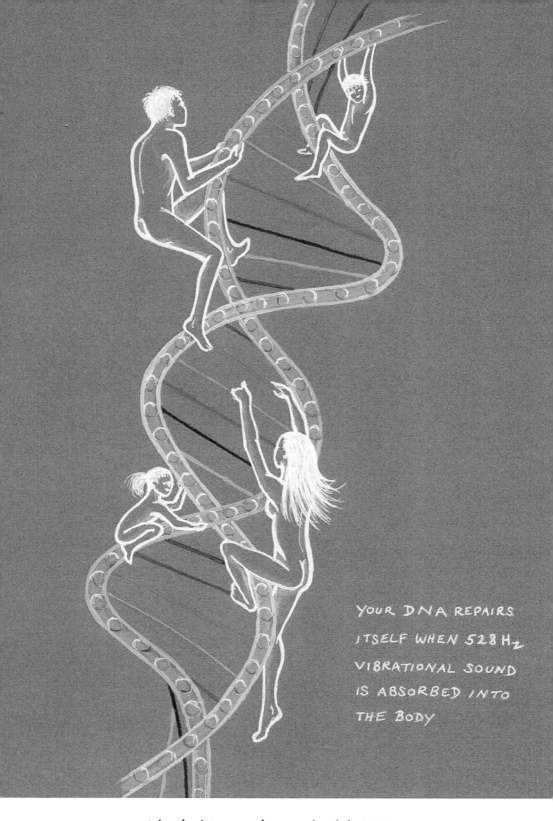

YOUR DNA REPAIRS
ITSELF WHEN 528 Hz
VIBRATIONAL SOUND
IS ABSORBED INTO
THE BODY

It's vital to repair your body's DNA

Chapter 7

Auras

Every new client I see has a Chakra and aura photograph taken. Our Chakras are invisible to the naked eye, and that's why I feel it is important to show a client what is going on from the outset. I'm able to give a verbal analysis on the findings of each Chakra and aura photograph taken. This process is repeated after every six hours of treatment, and these repeated photographs are a record of the client's progress and well-being, and are designed for them to keep throughout their journey.

An aura is a field of subtle, luminous radiation of light surrounding a person or object. It is said that all living things (including humans) and all objects manifest such an aura. While there are some people who are gifted enough to see other people's auras, most people are not that gifted. The depiction of such an aura often connotes with a person's demeanour and personality. Various writers associate various personality traits with the colours of different layers of the aura, and it has also been described as a map of the thoughts and feelings surrounding a person.

The aura of a person is also directly connected to the level of health of the person. A person is considered to be healthy in terms of physical vitality, mental clarity and emotional well-being as well as having a highly positive spiritual energy. So a person who is healthy at all these levels has a bigger and brighter aura, and vice-versa in the case of an unhealthy person.

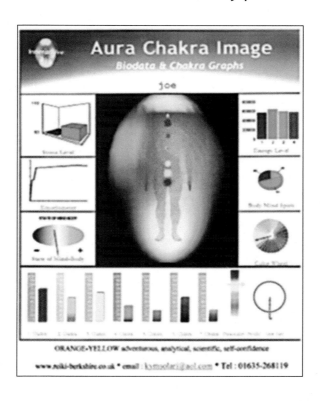

Chapter 8

Energies: The Future – The Now – The Past

How many of us can't wait to book another holiday whilst we're on the plane coming back from the one we've just had? That thought process is about you in that moment having a *desire for the future.*

How many of us have been desperate to stretch out a 24-hour day because we are enjoying what we are doing on that particular day? That's your conscious mind and self, *living in the now.*

How many of us have experiences and skeletons in our closets of past decisions and actions that we have made that we are desperate to forget, but cannot? The past can stick to us like Super Glue, and it is as damaging to our desire to move forward as black ice on the road while driving. On the other hand, some of us have lovely memories of the past that we desire to either relive or hold onto when the now becomes too overwhelming. This is the *fear of letting go of the past*, but we must do this to allow room for your future to evolve and happen.

I would like you all to imagine that your body is like the map of the UK, and that the weather is determined by jet streams and currents. As an example, if the jet streams and currents coming in from the Atlantic are free-flowing, we have beautiful sunshiny days. But if these currents are interrupted by turbulent winds coming from the east, then we can experience hail, wind, rain and even snow. Or we can also end up with just plain, stagnant and going nowhere days.

Now how does this all relate to the human body? And how do the currents relate to your past, present and future?

The inability to let go of the past becomes a solid dam blocking your future positive energy coming in. Therefore, you spend your life in a dead-end job you're not happy with or stay in a dead-end marriage that's going nowhere or even a dead-end friendship. You will eventually wake up everyday with a sense of loathing and hatred for yourself and others. Your desire to be in the present then becomes cloudy and unhealthy.

I need to be clear. Only an energy healer can move away and remove this stagnant energy to allow your present to be sharper and your future to come in. Living in the now and embracing your future makes every man, woman and child *happy, strong, confident* and *loving.*

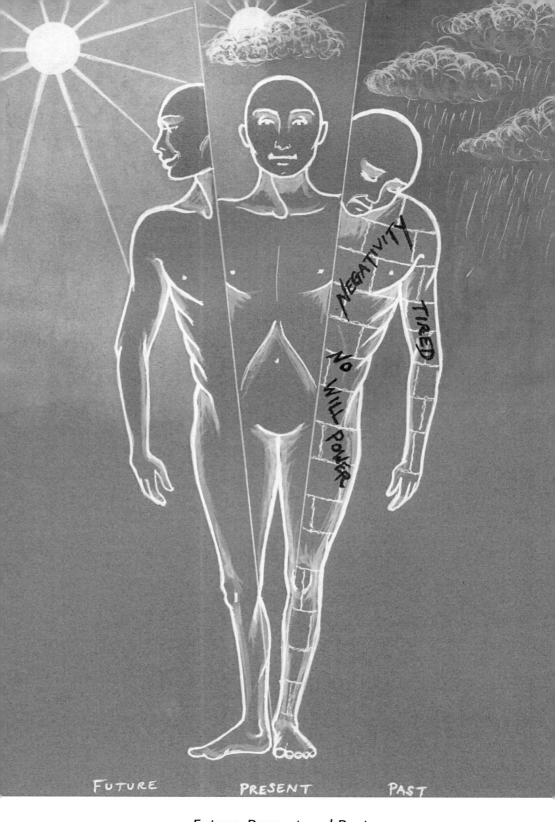

Future, Present and Past

Toxic relationships

These relationships can be with parents, siblings, friends, work colleagues, spouses and even with our own children. Most of us, at some point in our lives, have experienced the effects of being in a toxic relationship. These relationships are very difficult to rise up against because we never truly believe that somebody so close to us that we love and care about could or would be toxic.

These relationships can definitely put us on a very dark spiral of self-destruction. This may show itself in consuming too much alcohol, food, drug addiction and self-harming. There is no age limit on these kinds of relationships but sadly we allow them to go on for years, and years, and years. However, the one thing that we need to do is find the strength and power to re-work the relationship or to walk away for good. Most of us will wake up in the morning and refresh ourselves with a lovely hot cup of tea, coffee, or even a lovely hot chocolate. How many of us wake up longing to have a refreshing cup of de-icer with a splash of bleach, a dash of vinegar and a bit of rat poison sprinkled on top? Of course, nobody does, but this is what a toxic relationship tastes like. Seeing these toxic substances written down is thought-provoking. What happens when you push your feelings and resentments down into your body, because of what is happening to you, causes the clarity between you and the behaviour you are receiving, to decay within your Chakras and your own self-worth.

By the inability to unhook yourself from these relationships you are preventing and delaying beautiful, pure and loving relationships coming into your precious life. Through my work with clients I am for ever dismayed at how long they have put up with this devastating behaviour.

The recipient of this behaviour tends to be submissive and needy and have an overwhelming desire to be liked, loved and needed. These traits are also found in children as young as five years of age, so parents and teachers need to be observant and sensitive to this kind of bullying taking place right under their noses.

If we can all, in this 21st century, apply some of the ancient techniques highlighted in this book into our daily lives, we will all find that our awareness and wellness will very subtly steer us towards healthier and better human beings.

Chapter 9

Stress

Stress is an invisible killer, just like diabetes. It creeps up on you when you least expect it and it sticks to you in the same way that dried concrete would stick to steel rods when preparing the foundations of a suspension bridge. Men, women and children are all vessels for this debilitating illness. It is the biggest killer known to man, and triggers many physical illnesses like cancer, heart attacks, strokes, diabetes, infertility, IBS and OCD – just to name a few. In 2012, the leading cause of death was actually heart disease, which as we know is caused by stress.

Stress also triggers many mental illnesses and dependencies such as alcoholism, domestic violence, drug use, intolerances, affairs, suicides and eating disorders.

Keeping stress away from your physical and mental body is a responsibility that solely falls upon you, the individual, and not your GP. The above lists fall within all of our own control to not suffer from. Stress is something that can be eliminated by weekly/fortnightly or monthly visiting of various holistic services. I am also including children in this, as they are fragile, and also suffer from stress.

Below is a list of suggestions of well documented treatments that do reduce stress. Please find one that suits you, and stick with it!...

- Acupuncture

- Reflexology

- Homeopathy

- Aromatherapy

- Massage with essential oils

- Meditation

- Visiting a Reiki Practitioner or Master

- And of course – the best of all for your body, mind and soul – ME!

The treatments in this book you will have to pay for; after all, your well-being is your responsibility. What these regular visits may cost you is nothing compared to what could happen to you if you ignore your inner voice.

This is a quote my husband has stuck on his dressing room door:

"A good wife and good health are a man's best wealth."

And I have on my dressing room door:

"A good husband and good health are a woman's best wealth."

(In case you are having trouble figuring out the point, it is that **health** *rhymes with* **wealth***!)*

Many people depend too much on prescription drugs, when they really don't work. For example, I have treated many men and women who have been on antidepressants for years and they were no more forward than when they started. Pills will never work. They just make you even more depressed by making you lethargic, needy and dependent.

Really – what human being wants to feel like that?

We should all want to live our lives to the full and embrace our future head on with a stressless life.

This book is not going to prevent stress coming your way. But what I hope it will do is prevent you allowing it to take a hold on your body and mind, so it doesn't drastically affect your life and that of your family and friends.

Cancers, heart attacks, strokes, high blood pressure, diabetes, MS, ME, IBS, depression, insomnia, anorexia, infertility and many other health problems are all caused by individuals not listening to their bodies until one of the above occurs. The bespoke treatment that I offer will eliminate most of the above with commitment and dedication to your own personal desire to *regain flawless health*.

This is not a book about diminishing the role of our GPs, it's a book about you all thinking outside of the box:

"The greatest medicine of all is to teach people how not to need It."

Chapter 10

The Importance of Gifting Your Body Silence

The lyrics from The Tremeloes' song "Silence is Golden" are so apt.

Gifting your body silence is as important as gifting yourself a holiday. By giving ourselves silence, we turn our thoughts and focus inwards and gain the power we need to refuel our minds. We start to see the beauty within and focus on our dreams and desires.

Quieting the mind can happen after years of practising the art of meditation, by having a good night's sleep or simply whatever works for you. I have found that my mind is at its most quiet when I iron – and when I talk and think about ironing I salivate! I feel this happens because my body knows I'm going to put it into silent mode.

Everyone is different, so please take the time to study your own body's awareness of what makes you silent and what happens when you are in this silence. In this silence you can manifest your dreams and desires and let your true self be connected to your own flow of energy around you. When was the last time you sat in silence and heard the sound of your own breath and felt the stillness of your soul? If you are like most people it's probably been a while, or even never.

Children also need to learn the art of silence, as it will benefit them greatly as they get older. They need to understand that silence can be more energizing than anything and that it is accessible to them and us whenever we feel the need to connect with our soul self. This is something that mums and dads can do on a weekly basis with their children by sitting in a circle in the living room or all sitting at the kitchen table or on a car trip or journey. To begin with, sitting in silence for 5–10 minutes is enough, and you just build it up as the weeks go by. You will soon notice very quickly that your children, along with you, will be calm and serene.

As well as teaching our children the art of silence, they also need to learn the art of self-expression as early in their development as possible. This will allow them to express their feelings in a concise manner without prejudice and fear.

As an example, this can be done by having a "family talking circle" where a talking pole is passed to each family member in turn to express themselves on anything they want to talk about. No family member has the right to interrupt or speak unless they are holding the talking pole. This example can be done weekly, fortnightly or monthly to encourage all family members to open up their Throat Chakra.

This is an old Native American custom which enabled both young and old, within the tribe, to come together without prejudice or hierarchy. This allowed everyone's voice to be heard, with no one being of lesser importance than the others, regardless of age.

Chapter 11

The Benefits of a Good Night's Sleep

The benefits of owning and listening to my 528Hz healing CD will enable insomniacs to finally experience a good night's sleep. Even if you're not an insomniac, but wake up periodically throughout the night or just find it hard to catch a good night's sleep, then my CDs will benefit you greatly.

Sleep plays a vital role in your good health and well-being throughout your life. Getting enough quality sleep at the right times can help protect your mental health, physical health, quality of life and safety.

The way you feel while you're awake depends in part on what happens while you're sleeping. During sleep, your body is working to support healthy brain function and maintain your physical health as to help repair your heart and blood vessels, to prevent diseases such as heart disease, high blood pressure, diabetes and stokes.

The damage from sleep deficiency can occur in an instant, such as a car crash, or it can harm you over time. For example, ongoing sleep deficiencies can raise your risk for some chronic health problems. It can also affect how well you think, react, work, learn, cope with change, control your emotions and get along with others. However, sleep deficiency also has been linked to depression, suicide and risk-taking behaviour.

In children and teens, sleep helps to support growth and development. If they are sleep deficient then they may have problems getting along with others. They may feel angry and impulsive, have mood swings, feel sad or depressed or lack motivation. They also may have problems paying attention and they may get lower grades and feel stressed.

The best night's sleep can once again be achieved by listening to my healing CD.

Chapter 12

Dangers of Our Smartphones

In the 21st century we are all being seduced by the digital era of smartphones, iPads, Xboxes, and the latest high tech gadgets, all of which cost an absolute fortune. When Apple launches a new product, thousands of people wait in line for hours through the day and night just to buy these very expensive devices. We have become so dependent on these products that we will go to any lengths to own one.

We think nothing of spending upwards of £800 on a smartphone but we would not spend money on a lifesaving MRI, mammogram or a second opinion with a private consultant. Instead, we wait in line for months at a time for the overstretched, overburdened NHS to send us an appointment through. What is wrong with this picture?

Your health and well-being is your responsibility and where you choose to seek advice on this and the outcome, falls firmly within your choices and priorities.

GPs are seeing more and more people with Repetitive Strain Injury and back problems because we refuse to put these damn devices down. There was a time when if you went out for dinner there would be a warm buzz of conversations in the air, now there is predominantly silence with the occasional beeping of messages being sent and received.

The art of conversation is becoming an out of date, inconsequential thing to do. We should all be worried about this trend as we are encouraging the world to become a one- or two-syllable, robotic generation.

Our smartphone has become the most precious and cared for thing in our lives. We are stressed and panic-stricken when we have no way of re-charging our phones and because of this more and more entrepreneurs are coming up with the most ingenious ways of preventing our phones from running out of power. Everything from clothing and what we carry is being designed so we can plug ourselves in and re-charge our precious devices.

The average person checks their phone 110 times a day. During peak times this equates to once every six or seven seconds, with some users unlocking their devices up to 900 times over the course of a day. You would think from the above statistic that this would eliminate our frustration of not receiving a reply ASAP but I'm afraid to say that is not the case. Our frustration and stress levels are forever increasing when replies take longer than we expect. We have willingly given up our own personal power to these devices.

I do understand the importance of keeping in touch with family, friends and colleagues but I do feel the obsession is getting out of control.

Whilst Facebook and Twitter are a great way of keeping in touch with family and friends it can become a very dark and destructive tool when used to bully and groom.

Children as young as five years of age are now putting mobile phones down as their first and most desired gift for Christmas and birthdays.

I would like to encourage you all to have a fresh new look at your smartphone and imagine that the apps on your phone are actually major organs in your body.

I have highlighted **Facebook in red** as this relates to the Root Chakra and on an emotional level it is about feeling secure or insecure. Many of you I am sure have woken up after an evening out with friends to see unflattering photos of yourself that either you or a so-called friend has popped on Facebook. Regardless of who posted the pictures, this is a violation of your privacy and will immediately create mistrust, hurt and insecurity.

On a physical level this creates a "fight or flight" tendency and in some cases the need to have cursory sex to fill a void of loneliness and insecurity. Sadly this will often lead to urinary infections and venereal diseases.

If you find that you are addicted to Facebook it is a sign of you feeling insecure and needy, with an overwhelming desire to belong liked and loved. This need was planted within you from the moment you were born. I would like to suggest that the time you spend on Facebook, you spend in front of a mirror talking to yourself in a loving and uplifting way. No one can destroy you if you build your own strong loving foundation.

I have highlighted the **email icon in orange** as this relates to the Sacral Chakra. On an emotional level this relates to relationship issues, greed, creativity, power – i.e. your power or the lack of it. If you are unable to keep away from your emails please examine whether this app has power over you or you have the power over it: to read or not to read, WHO HOLDS THE POWER?

On a physical level this relates to prostate and cervical cancers, back and circulation problems.

If you find you are addicted to your email app, this is a sign that you felt powerless with the decisions in your infant and informative years.

I have highlighted the text message icon in yellow as this relates to the Solar Plexus Chakra. On an emotional level this is the desire to or not to communicate. For example if you are being hounded by a friend, work colleagues, your boss, siblings or parents, this will manifest itself in a physical form of eating disorders and IBS.

If you are addicted to this app please be aware of your toiletry pattern. Bloating around the stomach can be caused by your large and small intestines not being relaxed and therefore you are unable to have a bowel movement. In the old days our mothers and grandmothers used to spring clean the house ready for the onset of spring. This is something I feel is very useful with our friends. If we continually hold on to old, stale, sour relationships we are not creating any room for new vibrant friendships, so don't be afraid to spring clean: you will be surprised at who will enter your life.

I have highlighted the battery icon in green as it relates to the Heart Chakra. Whenever we touch our phones we automatically scroll our eyes over the "battery life" indicator. We sigh with relief when it shows 70%+ full and panic intensely when we see we are only 15+% full. We then rush to see what we have left opened that is running down the battery, or frantically look for our charger. It should be self-explanatory to all of you why I have popped a heart in this square – or maybe not!

The next time you reach for your phone and see that the battery is dangerously low I implore you all to step away from what you are doing and give your heart a little bit of TLC and rest your mind, body and soul for just 5 or 10 minutes. You will be surprised how much calm and clearer you will feel.

On an emotional level the heart relates to love, happiness, desires, sadness, grief, choices in love and career etc. On a physical level it relates to heart disease, angina, pneumonia, respiratory problems, etc. If you are addicted to your phone never losing its charge, I implore you to follow the above statement. As you only have one heart you need to protect and nurture it, just as we do these blasted devices.

I have highlighted the phone icon in blue as it relates to the Throat Chakra. On an emotional level this Chakra relates to speaking the truth, or not. This is a very under-used ability when talking on the phone as we all prefer to hide behind our statements, especially when we can blame misinterpreted comments as "Oh, it must have been predictive text." On a physical level more and more of us need to become more confident of speaking our truth as, especially in men, more and more throat and parathyroid cancers are being diagnosed.

I have highlighted the **camera icon in mauve** as this relates to our Third Eye Chakra. It is all about our dreams and inner knowing. Trust your intuition and you will not fall foul of stupidity. On an emotional level this is about open mindedness, acceptance, listening and seeing clearly.

On a physical level this highlights problems with teeth and gums, eye problems, the brain and nervous system. If you are addicted to this icon and you are not a professional photographer it highlights the desire to record everything you do and see, for in the past you may have been wrongly accused of being a liar.

I have highlighted the app store icon in white as this relates to the crown Chakra. This is about our desire for knowledge and a higher understanding of things. On an emotional level this relates to being spontaneous, valuing yourself and being free spirited.

On a physical level this relates to exhaustion, depression, psoriasis and alopecia. If you are addicted to this app you need to get out in the fresh air and not be such an introvert. Bring more fun into your life.

***

In this chapter I wanted to highlight the fact that if we took as much care and attention over our body's health and major organs as we do our "cannot do without" devices, we would be a happier, healthier society. We would be less of a burden on our NHS and doctors' surgeries.

Our GPs get a poor rap – we can never get an appointment, they have never got enough time, I was misdiagnosed... We hear these statements all the time from our family, friends and neighbours as well as in the media.

A general practitioner is someone with a loose and vague knowledge of diagnosis and treatments and therefore on consulting one's GP we should be mindful of the limitations of their expertise. This is why we have consultants and specialists. GPs are becoming increasingly overwhelmed by the pressure patients put upon them to assess and diagnose their symptoms correctly. Our beloved GPs are becoming patients themselves. We are being made aware of this by the numbers leaving the profession which results in surgeries closing.

The UK's general practitioners have little to no knowledge of alternative therapies and all the amazing benefits associated with them. Alternative therapies have been around since the 1800s and in Asia alternative therapy is the first port of call for anyone feeling unwell. Most of the oldest people in the world come from this continent. To my knowledge very few doctors in the UK will suggest alternative therapies. Sadly our GPs are becoming more and more like drug barons, as the pharmaceutical companies have a huge commercial interest in a drug-dependent society.

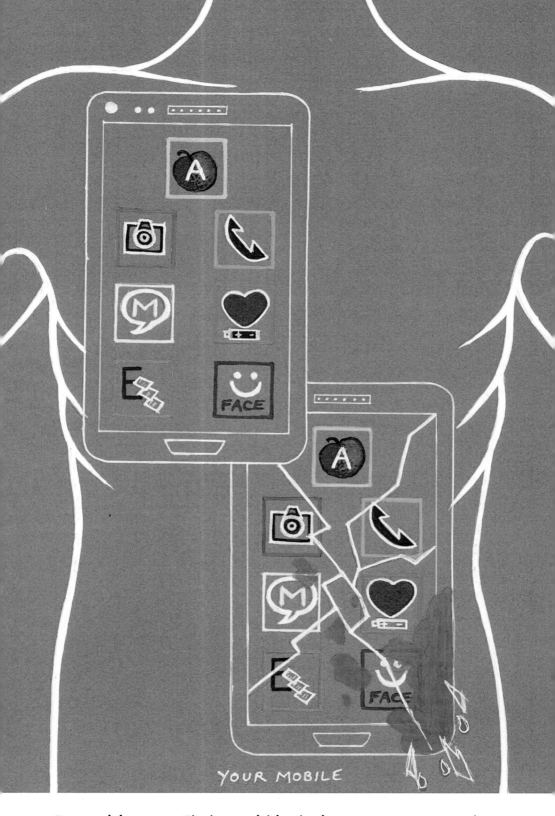

YOUR MOBILE

Recognizing your Chakras within the icons on your smartphone

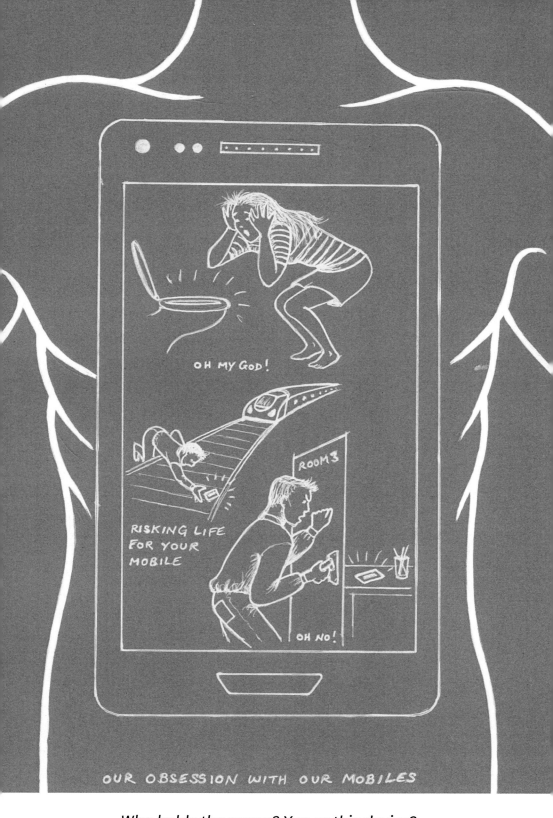

Who holds the power? You or this device?

Chapter 13

Newborns and Children

As parents there are three important things we must provide for our children:

1 A loving home and security.

2 A good education.

3 Making them see that their Health is their only Wealth.

I appreciate that for many parents out there, this has not been on their radar as much as it should. All life is precious, but it hits a totally different level when you, as parents, are dealing with a sick child.

We are all familiar with the phrase:

"My child should be burying me and not me burying my child."

The increase in children's cancers, diabetes, obesity and ADHD is soaring out of control. This does not have to be the case. I have written this chapter especially for you, the parents out there who are looking for a new approach to your child's health, and I hope it will raise awareness and provoke discussion.

As explained in Chapter 5 (page 56), your child is born with a pure symphony which is influenced by the symphony of those around them. Your child's soul energy field (aura) is also open and vulnerable to the atmosphere surrounding them. The aura is continually building throughout their life, and all of one's life experiences can be found there – good or bad.

Whether things are out in the open or not, your child senses what's going on between his/her parents and this behaviour from the parents will determine temperament, fears, fantasies, or illnesses of the child, which will manifest as they grow older into adulthood and will ricochet into their own marital life and their newly born children.

For example, if a child was conceived to keep the marriage alive, the child will sense the underlying current of unhappiness and turmoil between his/ her parents and will subconsciously be aware of the huge burden that has been placed upon such small shoulders. Hence, this child will grow up with insecurity issues and will have a need to constantly overachieve throughout their life to be liked and loved.

Parents must be aware that whilst in the womb their baby has been cocooned and protected in its own subconscious mind as well as feeling warm, cozy and protected in its own liquid of peace and harmony. Once born, the little body and mind is shocked into the reality of constant noise, cries, smells and blinding lights. No wonder the little body goes into lockdown.

This happens as a protection mechanism, so if your child suffers from colic, or refuses to eat or sleep, remember it's their survival mechanism kicking in. All parents need to do is create the same cozy, dim lighted and noise free protective environment like the baby had in the womb. This way, the Chakras and his/her mental state will develop at a calm and smooth rate. One way to ensure this is by committing to regular sessions and by playing my 528Hz healing CD throughout pregnancy and throughout all sleep times.

This highlights the importance of the environment we create at home and at work, what we do in our lives and how it has a direct impact on our Chakras and aura. This relates to how we are as a human being and the illnesses that will occur throughout our life.

All of the information found on Chapter 2 relates directly to your child's health and wellbeing, throughout their lives.

I feel it's important that all parents should have knowledge of the frequency that best suits their newborn child.

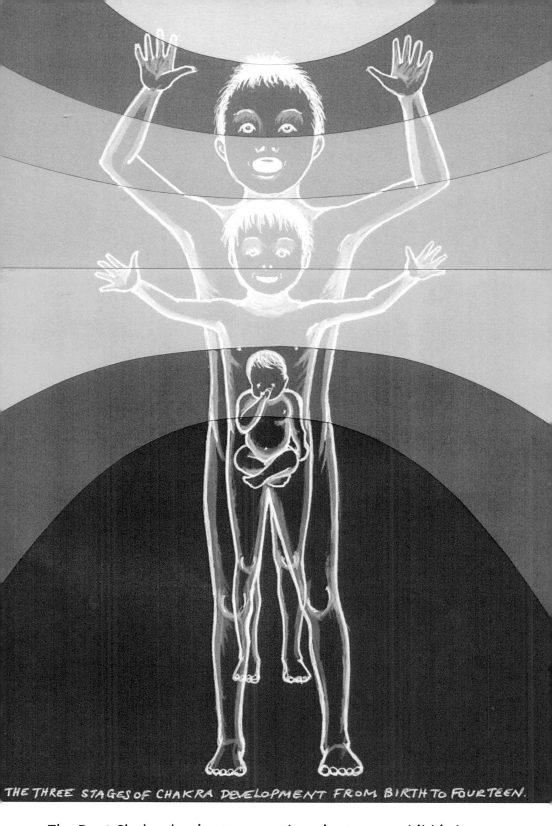

THE THREE STAGES OF CHAKRA DEVELOPMENT FROM BIRTH TO FOURTEEN.

The Root Chakra begins to open the minute your child is born

Once a child is born, its surroundings and noise will influence his/her new soul's energy field (the aura). Each event adds a little colour to the aura and enhances its individuality. The aura is continually building throughout life, and all of one's life experiences can be found there – good or bad. Your child's energy field is entirely open and vulnerable to the atmosphere in which he/she lives.

Chapter 14

Our Beloved Pets

Our beloved pets have Chakras and auras too and must be loved, cared and protected just like newborn babies.

For behavioural problems that may be occurring in our pets, Reiki is the perfect way of healing as it can be practiced with the pet at any distance and be adapted to suit the personal need of the pet. There is virtually no problem or circumstance that cannot be treated effectively by Reiki and vibrational sound healing, so once again, purchasing my 528Hz healing CD would be of great benefit for your pets.

For example, my beautiful toy poodles Tifo and Piccio came into my home at 9½ weeks old. They would go to sleep every night listening to my healing CD cuddled around my body on my bed. They also spend their day in my healing studio with me, again being exposed to vibrational sound and my healing bowls. They are beautifully calm, well-tempered angels. I have had toy poodles for over 25 years and I can say without a word of a lie that all of my poodles have passed into spirit well into their 16th and 17th year.

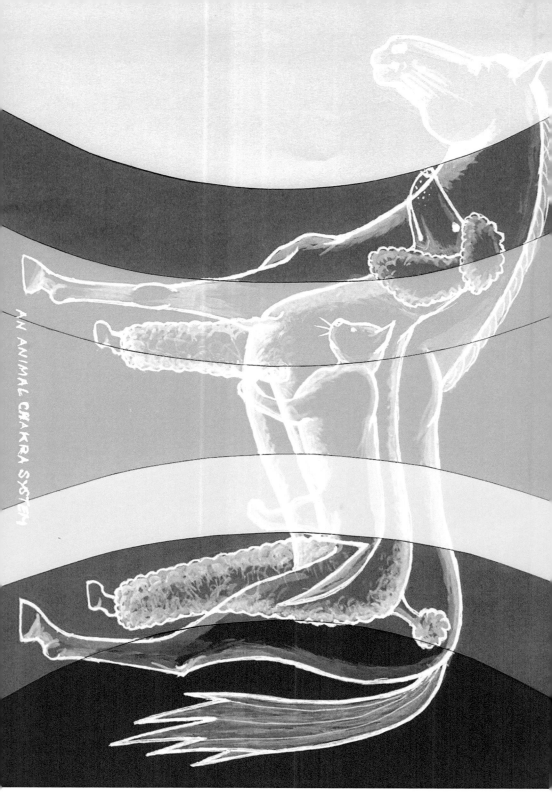

AN ANIMAL CHAKRA SYSTEM

Yes, your animals have Chakras too!

Chapter 15

To Have or Not to Have...

When you, or a family member, has been given the devastating news that cancer is alive and thriving in what you thought was your healthy body, it is overwhelmingly hard to process. Within moments of receiving this news you are thrust into the world of clinicians' jargon, which you are, at this time, unable to process.

We have all been conditioned to believe that someone who has cancer is going to pass away and the prospect of this is overwhelmingly numbing and frightening. But this does not have to be the case. It is my strong belief that if you combine the advice of your clinicians with a strong holistic approach you have a much better chance of coming through the other side of this most terrifying news.

As someone who has worked primarily with cancer patients for over a decade and a half, I can heart-warmingly say that my clients, who hold my type of holistic healing as fundamental to their well-being throughout, have sailed through the clinical onslaught on their bodies.

Please don't expect your oncologist, or their team, to embrace or even acknowledge your decision to have this holistic approach simultaneously whilst undergoing their clinical ideology. Few physicians have hands-on experience delivering non-drug treatments that actually helps people to recover their health.

What a lot of people fail to realise is that cancer thrives in a body where the body's own immune system has been weakened and stripped out by chemotherapy and radiation. My treatment, with the introduction of the 528Hz DNA bowl, over time, regenerates the body's dead immune system, which enables a cancer patient to fight back at the core of the disease.

Time and time again my clients report back to me on how their hospital appointment with their oncologist has gone. Even when their oncologist is surprisingly struck by the incredible progress my client has made, they have shown no interest in exploring what else this patient may have been doing to supplement and encourage their wellbeing, which, time and time again, shows up on their follow-up blood tests and scans. This lack of interest on the part of their oncologist and their team has a very negative and dismissive effect on my clients, their cancer patients.

There was a 12-year study published in 1994 in the United States that looked at adult cancers. They did a MEDA analysis of all the people around the world who developed adult cancers, for 12 years, and were treated with chemotherapy and they looked at the results and published the results in the journal of clinical oncology. In the results 97% of the time chemotherapy does not work, so why is it used?

I think it is about time the oncologists got their heads out of the big pharmaceutical companies' ass and attended one of my seminars. They can hear and see for themselves how vitally important it is, for their patients to have the holistic approach side by side with chemotherapy and radiation. My bespoke treatment rebuilds a patient's immune system, their mental and emotional health.

People are confused and unsure whether or not to partake in the treatment described in this book that I offer, due to their own religious beliefs and doctrines. I would like to make it crystal clear that whatever spiritual or religious beliefs you have (or do not have), healing *will* occur if you completely surrender to the universal energy that surrounds us all and trust the healer who is the channel for this energy. As a healer, I pray more in a day than most people would do in a year. I am extremely religious and divinely spiritual and that is my personal belief as to why I achieve the results that I do. But I must emphasize that it does not matter whether you are a religious person or not, and if you are, then it does not matter which religion you follow, as the healer's energy will still heal you.

Each individual that has benefited from my treatment humbles me beyond words. Cancer patients often come after years of chemotherapy and deadly radiation and all have startling journeys to tell on how these conventional medicines are rapidly killing every cell in their body. Finally, the killing of their cells ends in my treatment room and the repairing of their body can begin.

Appendix

Testimonials

On the following pages are amazing and totally true stories from a number of my patients, all of whom would be willing to defend this journey of healing and share it with anyone who is contemplating coming to see me.

Testimonial 1 (2007): Mike Rowe

The 1st of November 2007. The most important day of my life was the day I first met Kimberly.

One week prior to this life changing day, I had been diagnosed with a cancerous tumour on the base of my tongue and a secondary tumour on the floor of my mouth that looked like I had swallowed a boiled egg. The oncologist treating me told me that to remove my cancer I would need a 15-hour operation to remove the tumours and all the glands in my neck where smaller tumours were present.

The operation would require sawing through the bottom of my jaw and removing the entire left section of my face, as well as potentially leaving me with stroke-like symptoms if they accidentally cut the nerves to certain parts of my body. I was also looking at being fitted with a Tracheotomy and I would have been fed through a peg in my belly button. Reconstructive surgery would take place when the area was suitable for reforming. I was also told I would be in intensive Care for at least two weeks. This would then be followed by radiotherapy and chemotherapy. Having gone through all of this I would then receive several years of physiotherapy to learn how to speak and eat again.

Needless to say my family and I feared for my life and seeing my wife and boys so devastated broke my heart even more, as I felt I had let them all down terribly.

Fate, however, had a different journey in mind for me. I was blown away with what was to follow.

On October the 29th my wife Lyn called her reflexologist Gill who was into crystal stone healing to ask what crystal I should wear around my neck for healing and protection. Gill told my wife she would have a look in her healing book for the right crystal while she waited on the end of the phone. The answer Gill gave my wife was not the name of a crystal, but the name of a healer, Kimberley Solari, that Gill had met the previous day to talk about her becoming Reiki attuned by Kimberley. My wife trusted Gill and promptly called Kimberley. After the pleasantries of introduction, Kimberley passed the phone onto one of her cancer patients to chat with my wife about the importance of making an appointment to see Kimberley and how life changing it would be. We then arranged an appointment to meet with Kimberley on 1 November 2007.

On meeting Kimberley for the first time, my wife and I were given a completely new outlook on the future which up until then had been destroyed by the news of my cancer and the pre-conceived notion of death that followed.

As you can imagine my wife and I were extremely anxious and emotional and didn't know what to expect on arriving at Kimberley's healing room in the village of Headley, Berkshire. On entering, my wife and I instantaneously felt calm and relaxed for the first time since I was diagnosed. We were aware that we were in the presence of someone special. Kimberley asked me to explain what was wrong with me and what the recommended plan of action from my oncologist was. After telling her, Kimberley smiled and then gave me overwhelming evidence of my grandfather's and mother's presence who are both in spirit.

Kimberley explained that she was a Reiki Master and Vibrational Sound Practitioner and that her treatment would last for approximately one hour and she would be using quartz crystal healing bowls as well as Life Force energy (Reiki). I immediately booked a course of sessions.

Kimberley's treatment was incredibly powerful. I could feel the Life Force energy going into my whole body from her hands, as well as the vortex of vibrational energy from the different vibrational healing bowls that she uses. Kimberley can also pick up and interpret other energies within the room and told me that my mother was insisting that I seek a second opinion. At first I ignored the messages, but the more I ignored them, the more Mum kept giving me the same message until finally I acted upon her advice. I went to a different hospital and got a second opinion, convinced that the recommended treatment and operation would be the outcome. How wrong was I? I could not believe it when the surgeon at the second hospital told me I did not need the invasive and life-disfiguring surgery and that he could cure my cancer with radiation and chemotherapy alone. My mother was right; I was not going to have the supposedly life-saving operation that would disfigure me for life. My operation date was looming but I cancelled it straight away and decided to follow the advice of my Mum and the second hospital.

Lyn and I broke down in tears of joy when we left the second hospital after their opinion, as the messages that we had received from spirit had turned out to be true. It was amazing! But more was to follow.

I continued to have Kimberley's treatment on a daily basis as the effect on my wife and me was truly amazing. It put us in a stress-free state of mind and totally relaxed us, despite what I had been diagnosed with. We truly believed that Kimberley's treatment was helping to destroy my cancer, not only in a physical way but mentally and emotionally as well along with the feedback from spirit.

Having received 6 weeks of Reiki and vibrational sound treatment from Kimberley and only one course of chemotherapy, I received another mind blowing message from my mother in spirit, telling me through Kimberley:

'Your tumour has gone and you are cancer-free.'

Can you imagine my response! I thought Kimberley was out of her mind, and she was only telling me what I wanted to hear, but she was adamant about the message as it came from my mother. That very evening I was sat at home relaxing and watching television and mulling over in my mind the message when the phone rang. It was one of my oncologists from the second hospital. She rang to tell me that she had received the results of my recent MRI scan, and that strangely they could no longer see the tumour on my tongue. (I nearly died from shock and surprise!!) I proceeded to tell her that I already knew this as I had been told only hours before by my mother who was in spirit. She was obviously amazed by what I had told her and she wanted to know more. The conversation lasted for hours.

My journey continued and through choice, Lyn and I continued to go through radiation (as a belt and braces procedure). I was sorely tempted not to though, as my mother repeatedly tried to stop me as she said I did not need it.

I am now seven years on from my first diagnosis and I have been totally CANCER FREE for 6½ years with my handsome face still completely intact. I am leading an entirely normal life, enjoying every day that I have been blessed with. I still receive Reiki from Kimberley on a weekly basis as I feel it keeps me calm and relaxed and of course I never know what feedback I might get from my relatives in the spirit world.

Lyn and I cannot thank Kimberley enough for her wonderful healing, love and encouragement and the help that she gave us both through the most traumatic and most pleasurable journey of our lives.

Testimonial 1 (2007): Lyn Rowe's Thankfulness

When Mike was diagnosed with throat cancer my whole world fell apart AGAIN.

Sixteen years ago I lost my beloved sister to cancer and all I ever wonder is how different things could have been for all of us if I had known Kimberley then. I would not have my life crumble for the second time, which is why I was not going to sit back and lose Mike without a fight. Only it wasn't a fight; just a different journey.

Only by chance, or call it fate, did we find Kimberley through Gill. This was to be a journey for the whole family that would change our lives. From the first day after Kimberley's healing we both felt so different, so strong, confident and calm. Were we really fighting a battle against cancer? It never really felt that way!!

Our journey was unbelievable. Not only were the Reiki and the vibrational healing bowls very special and powerful, but we were also guided by spiritual feedback from loved ones. By being in the Reiki room while Mike was having his healing, it gave me such strength and a calmness that I had never experienced before. One thing that I will always remember is the amazing aroma Kimberley has in her room. This is achieved by not only burning incense sticks but also by her unique and bespoke healing oils that she blends herself.

I was a changed woman! My husband, who was the love of my life and my soul-mate, had cancer. But never did it once feel like I was going to lose him. Being a very anxious person since losing my sister to cancer, I always fear the worst of any situation, but Mike was going to be fine and live a long life; after all, his granddad in spirit told us so on our very first meeting with Kimberley. We had so much spiritual feedback, it was just amazing.

Just one example of this was when I had a private moment with my Dad one morning where I kissed his picture three times before leaving the house for Mike's healing treatment with Kimberley. To my utter surprise, after Mike's healing session that day, my Dad came through for me via Kimberley with a message to thank me for the lovely kisses. Who else knew that other than me?? Wow – Amazing!

Mike has been in remission for 6½ years and we both feel so blessed that our two sons have their Dad healthy and well. We both still go for regular healing sessions and life is just great. No stress. No anxiety. Perfect!

In April of 2010, my wife and I decided to go on a vegan diet and I was losing weight steadily. Then it seemed as though overnight I became gaunt and unhealthy looking. A routine blood test in September 2010 showed that I had an elevated calcium level. My GP believed that the problem was not my change in diet, but could be a tumour growth on one of my parathyroid glands. This often occurs when there is a certain elevated calcium level. Normally these types of tumours are benign and a simple minimally invasive procedure is performed to remove the tumour. I had two different scans that confirmed that it was indeed a tumour on one of my parathyroid glands and I immediately planned to have it removed.

I was referred to an endocrine surgeon who once again confirmed that tumours like this are 99.9% benign. The day of my surgery was routine. I signed the consent form in front of my wife and was duly taken down to the operating theatre. Moments into the procedure my surgeon left the room to tell my wife that my tumour was in fact cancerous.

Once back in the theatre, my surgeon removed the tumour which was 10.5cm which meant my thyroid had to also be removed. Once out and placed in a kidney dish, everyone in the theatre was amazed to see that the removed tumour was in fact crystallized; something they had never seen before. This meant that the surrounding tissues and lymph nodes were not affected by the cancer due to the amazing crystallization. This also meant that I needed no further treatment of any kind and that he would check me again in one year. He also made it very clear that in all his years of removing this type of tumour, he has never experienced a totally crystallized tumour which had prevented the cancer from spreading to other areas of my body.

I truly believe my tumour became crystallized due to my regular, once-a-week vibrational sound healing sessions from Kimberley who is a Reiki Master and Vibrational Sound Practitioner. Kimberley has developed a treatment combining Reiki and sound energy using quartz crystal healing bowls. I have found the treatment to be extremely soothing and relaxing and I could always feel the vibrations from the bowls penetrating my body with terrific sensation.

Its theses vibrations that I feel, in my case, actually helped crystallize the tumour and this crystallization stopped the cancer from spreading. I am totally sold on the power of vibrational healing bowls to actually enhance the well-being of people with all types of different ailments, both physical and mental.

I consider myself to be the luckiest man in the world.

On 1 November 2011, I was diagnosed with myeloma; a form of bone cancer. My power protein levels were staggeringly high, at around the 6000 mark. I was put straight onto a six-month medication of chemotherapy tablets steroids and some viral infection tablets called Acyclovir. All this medication and all of the pressure of having cancer and whether or not I would survive to see my children get married, play with my grandchildren, and of course, be here for my wonderful and loving wife, was causing me so much stress and strain.

Out shopping one day I bumped into Mike and Lyn Rowe, friends of mine, and they asked how my wife and I were doing. I briefly told them of my myeloma and they both recommended that I go and see a lady called Kimberley as she had helped this couple through their own cancer journey. I regrettably dismissed this recommendation as so many other things were going on in my head. I just left it. This was a very bad move on my part.

After the six months of treatment my protein levels were not reducing, so in May 2012, my doctor offered me autologous stem cell replacement therapy hoping it would give me nine years in remission. This to me was a wonderful opportunity so my wife and I agreed to go ahead.

So on 13 May 2012, at Churchill Hospital, I then had my own stem cells removed and then underwent a very harsh treatment of chemotherapy. This was to clear my body of as many myeloma-affected bone marrow cells as possible (known as conditioning), and then replacing them using my own clean stem cells (called engraftment). I was then put

*on Acyclovir. After a few weeks of recovery at home my life
started to get back to normal. I was asked to return to the
hospital for a routine blood test, where unfortunately I was
told that the myeloma had returned, now with a protein level
of 4000. I was then told I needed to be put on even more
medication of Velcade (chemotherapy) injections weekly for
six months. At this point I was so worried and troubled. My
life felt like it was crumbling to pieces.*

*Wondering what to do next, I remembered that brief
encounter whilst out shopping and decided to drive round to
Mike and Lyn's home and asked for Kimberley's details. Once
again, discussing it fully with my wife, we agreed to contact
Kimberley, and my true journey to recovery started.*

*I booked my first session with Kimberley in July, and after
that first treatment I felt so much more relaxed and at
ease that I was being given a helping hand on this terrible
journey of mine. I then continued having sessions with
Kimberley once every week and thankfully my protein levels
reduced from 4000 to 90.*

*My doctors were amazed at my dramatic turnaround to good
health, so much so, that on a routine visit I was offered a
bone marrow transplant. Shocked and surprised at this
amazing opportunity, I grabbed it with both hands. As you
can appreciate transplants do not happen overnight, and
they are very complicated procedures. However, I stayed
relaxed and calm as I was still having Kimberley's amazing
treatment and my life was fully back to normal.*

*I underwent the bone marrow transplant in 2013 and once
again my doctors were amazed at how my body responded
to the graft, and a five-week stay in hospital was reduced
to three as I was doing so well, and my protein levels were*

reduced to 72. The first thing I did on being released from hospital was to resume my once-a-week treatments with Kimberley. The medication I was put on after the transplant was Acyclovir, Cyclosporine and Cotrimoxazol and I was also taking Omeprazole for my high acid count and Penicillin to protect my spleen. But I was on these two treatments before I was diagnosed anyway, so I have come a long, long way! From the minute I walked into Kimberley's amazing treatment room my life has been completely transformed from having no hope of recovering, to my protein levels coming down and receiving the bone marrow transplant.

On a recent routine check-up, I have been told by my doctor, Dr Andy Remtikett, that my levels are excellent and he would like to offer me a top up of bone marrow from the donor, on Tuesday 17 June 2014, in a bid to reduce my protein levels to 40. He could not be happier for me. It is extremely rare to see a patient go from where I started to where I am today, and he is so shocked and amazed by my continued progression of amazingly good health.

I am quite an old-fashioned chap and the thought of going to see an alternative therapist would never have entered my mind; now, however, my whole outlook on this very supportive and non-invasive treatment has changed. Regrettably, I did not inform my oncologist that I was having Reiki and vibrational sound treatment with Kimberley as I thought he may dismiss me from under his care. I feel it's now too late as I am almost at the end of my journey back into good health and that is the reason why I want my case study to be in Kimberley's book. I hope that this testimonial will encourage all the men out there to embrace this treatment and I would wholeheartedly recommend it to anyone and everyone going through – not just cancer – but anything you are struggling with in your life.

My whole family and I are forever indebted to Kimberley, not just for her amazing and powerful treatment, but also for her tremendous love and support.

You can't NOT try it!

My 10 year old daughter became ill with sepsis neutropenia (a weak immune system) and thrombocytopenia (low number of platelets so excessive bleeding occurs) at the beginning of January 2013. The cause was never identified, except the hospital doctors decided it was probably a secondary infection to glandular fever. Her body mass loss exceeded the hospital's dietician scale, as she lost over a third of her weight, weighing approximately four stone. For months, she was unable to eat without nausea, drinking became increasingly difficult and she was unable to walk without pain or hold herself upright – so had to use a wheelchair or be carried everywhere. She was then diagnosed with CFS (chronic fatigue syndrome)/ME.

Anyway, it was recommended that we see a Reiki Master and thankfully we found Kimberley and got more than we bargained for. Her experience and healing power was beyond our wildest dreams. With one's child, we only ever wanted the very best treatment and practitioner that we could find and Kimberley was the one.

Kimberley uses a combination of vibrational sound, by using the quartz crystal healing bowls and Life Force energy (Reiki) as a treatment. As an electrical/electronic engineer, I thought the ingenious principle behind the combined treatments made complete sense (quantum theory); relaxing the body to make it receptive and then using a variety of bowls which vibrate at different hertz, thus, replicating the hertz in various parts of the body in which they are meant to be vibrating; what's more, allowing the body to heal itself.

After each treatment my daughter said she felt well and had more energy. After one of her treatments, whilst Kimberley was performing Reiki, Sophie woke suddenly and was looking at her feet. She said she saw Jesus. Interestingly, Sophie said that even though she has never seen a picture of Jesus or even looked at a Bible, she just knew it was him. That was all she had to say.

*There and then, I knew something very extraordinary had taken place during Sophie's healing session that day. We were told by our doctor that my daughter would be in a wheelchair for about three years, but it turned out to be **just a few weeks**. Her consultant at Bath Hospital has described her recovery as **'remarkable'** and she is now in full time school and just starting to take part in sports. She is enjoying life to the full and I truly believe that this would not have been possible if we hadn't have been blessed in finding Kimberley and her **exceptional and innovative combined treatment.***

Testimonial 5 (2013–14): Joe Thompson

My name is Joe Thompson. I am a 25 year old professional footballer. In 2013, I was playing for Tranmere Rovers. Within weeks of the new season starting, I just couldn't shake my flu-type symptoms, no matter what the club and I tried.
So in October the club doctors suggested I have a routine blood test, which I was happy to do. The club and I were not expecting anything unforeseen to be detected, so you can imagine our shock when the results of the blood tests and a minor biopsy came back showing that I had stage 3s non-sclerosing Hodgkin's lymphoma. The club spent no time in getting me to see a specialist in Liverpool, where more blood tests and scans were done and it did indeed confirm that I was in the advanced stage of Hodgkin's lymphoma.

My professor at the Murrayfield hospital, Wirral, explained that my playing days for the rest of the season of 2013 were over. Driving home from the hospital was the most surreal and scared I had ever been. On arriving home, I sat down and told my beautiful girlfriend Chantelle of the results. After a period of hugging and crying, our one year old daughter became sensitive to the upsetting atmosphere and began crying also. Focusing our attention on our beautiful daughter, we both dried our eyes and let the news sink in, and from somewhere deep inside us we knew I would get through this, but how? We had no idea. All we knew was that we needed help.

A few days passed and my manager at Tranmere told my teammates that I would be missing for the rest of the season at least, due to the results from my blood tests and biopsy that confirmed I had a rare form of cancer; Hodgkin's lymphoma. A few days later, with my permission, Tranmere broke the news publicly. As you can imagine, the minute the news broke, the inbox on my phone was bursting with encouraging voicemails and texts from teammates and others, all wishing me well. With my emotions still raw, I wasn't in the mood to talk much to anyone but one call in particular from my team mate James Rowe inspired me to call him back. James told me about a lady called Kimberley who had worked miracles on his dad when he was diagnosed with cancer in 2007. James insisted I give this lady a call, and more importantly, get my arse off the couch and drive the 400 miles round trip to go and see her. My doctors hadn't come up with a treatment plan yet, so what did I have to lose?

I then met James' mum and dad at Tranmeres' next game, where they could not be more forceful in telling me that I had to go and see Kimberley.

So the following week, Chantelle and I, along with our beautiful daughter Lula-Lily, drove four hours from Manchester to Wantage where we stayed with James' parents. The very next day, we drove to Newbury to meet Kimberley and on arrival we immediately felt in safe hands. Kimberley spent a good two hours explaining to me and Chantelle that her innovative vibrational healing treatment would work hand in hand with any additional treatment, such as chemotherapy, to help to rid my body of this cancer and re-build a healthier me. I started my journey into vibrational healing there and then.

The plan was that we would stay at Mike and Lynn Rowe's home and I would have the short drive to Kimberley's, where I would have four to five hours of treatment a week. Just after four hours of treatment, I noticed that my cancerous symptoms suddenly subsided. We were amazed. It reinforced my belief that with Kimberley and chemotherapy I would be cured.

My doctors in Liverpool suggested that as I lived in Manchester, it may be more beneficial if I were to see a consultant in Manchester, and as luck would have it, I was referred to Professor John Radford, a Professor of Medical Oncology/Honorary Consultant, at the Christie Hospital, who was doing clinical trials with a drug called Echelon 1. This would be given to me once a fortnight for six months. Dr Radford and his staff made it fully clear that the side-effects of this drug and any other kind of chemotherapy would be severe. Although I did feel a few side-effects, I knew that Kimberley's treatment was helping me drastically with these as well.

I would like to emphasize that I had had 12–16 hours of Kimberley's treatment prior to starting with this trial drug. The joy of being on a trial drug means that you undertake more frequent blood tests and scans than normal. I am happy to tell you that within only two months of starting the treatment, my bloods were coming back, showing that I was negative to the strain of Hodgkin's lymphoma. Dr Redford was keen to point out that this was an extremely positive sign going forward. However, there was a long road ahead. To my amazement, each blood test was showing the same amazing results that I was indeed staying negative to the strain of Hodgkin's lymphoma, and moreover, four months into the trial, there were no tumours visible in my body. I need to point out that before I started with Kimberley and Echelon, I had numerous tumours in my neck, a larger mass down my sternum and two tumours in my spleen.

On 16 July 2014, after nine months of Kimberley's vibrational sound treatment and six months of Echelon 1, I was given the most amazing news that I was in complete remission.

Kimberley, my professor and I were over the moon. Words could not describe what it means to me and my family that I am healthy and strong again. I am in the process of building up my body strength to return to the career that I love and that is playing football and if I am allowed another dream – it would be to one day play for England.

I deeply believe that without Kimberley's vibrational healing I may have not survived, so to her I am truly grateful!

Testimonial 5 (2013–14): Chantelle's thankfulness

When my partner was first diagnosed with cancer I felt like our world had ended. It was such a scary time for me and my family. I cannot thank Kimberley enough for what she has done for Joe. I believe that her bespoke Reiki and vibrational sound sessions have not only helped to shrink his tumours, but also helped greatly with the side-effects of the chemotherapy. Kimberley was very forceful in explaining that I too would benefit from having a session now and again to help with the stress and pressure of having the man that you love being diagnosed with such a very scary disease like cancer. The only way I can describe her treatment is that it is magical and wonderful. One of the things that I will remember for ever will be the beautiful smells in Kimberley's healing room. I cannot stress to people enough how Kimberley and her bespoke treatment helped us through the toughest time of our lives.

I will be forever grateful.

Testimonial 6 (2014–15): Helen Hodgkinson

Most stories about cancer begin with the day of diagnosis. Today is 6 May 2015 and my daughter Isobel, who is nine, has cancer: she has been diagnosed for nearly six months now and this is the story of our life, well at least for the last few months and as we are beginning to learn will be part of our future.

Most stories begin with how devastating the situation is and yep, that is true but there are two parts to this story, an emotional and a medical one. Kimberley, or as she is known in our house "the angel healer", has had a part to play in both. We stand today together as a family supporting Isobel because of her, but that is part of the tale, Isobel's current position and the way she has handled her treatment and has fought her cancer has much to do with the vibrational healing Kimberley has developed.

So finally going back to November 2014, the 12th to be precise and her ninth birthday. We were told the devastating news that Isobel had cancer, originally diagnosed with a Ewing's sarcoma which was later re diagnosed as a non-Hodgkin's B cell lymphoma. It began with pain in her shoulder for which she had physiotherapy. During this a lump was discovered and whilst investigations were underway a further visible lump appeared in her eye, rendering her blind. On internal investigation another three tumours were found on her knee, breast plate and elbow.

In this crazy world of paediatric oncology you meet many people each with a traumatic tale to tell. Kimberley was recommended to us by another family whom she was also treating, how they described what Kimberley did was "your

*medics are being medics and Kimberley is a great healer,
helping all that they do". On 9 December 2014 all of the
family visited Kimberly including our other children Ruby (7)
and Ted (5). There are no words to describe how we arrived
that day: Isobel was ill and we were broken. That was the
first day that Kimberley began to repair this family and to fix
Isobel. It's important to remember at this point Isobel had
not even started chemo yet.*

*During that visit where we all participated in Kimberley's
healing we started the journey to where we are today. The
first thing Kimberley told us, she will be fine, the only person
still to have said this to us. I cannot tell you what that does
for you as a family when you believe all is lost. And for the
first time we felt in safe hands and able to conquer this
battle.*

*Chemo started three days later, this is the first visible sign
we had of the effect of vibrational therapy. Isobel's tumour
in her eye had reduced, this was after only two treatments,
this was confirmed by her medical team and her tumours
have continued to reduce as she has continued to be
treated.*

*The effect on the tumours is clear, a combination of the
medical treatment and vibrational healing has meant
Isobel is fast on her way to recovery, we are only a quarter
of the way through her medical treatment and she is doing
so incredibly well. Everybody in her care package is really
pleased with her progress*

*But added to this is how well she has coped with the
treatment regime which is brutal for adults – and for a nine
year old, frankly it is disgusting. But she fares so much
better than others in her position, her side-effects are*

minimal, she still attends school, she sees her friends and in the last three weeks has been playing cricket which is unheard of. This is down to vibrational healing.

We see Kimberley three times a week, Isobel asks to go and never refuses, for me that is testament in itself. There is no doubt Isobel would not be where she is without her, but she also has helped us as a family, healing our scars, keeping us together and making sure we can stitch together our past, present and future. We all need this and truly would not have survived without it.

I bring many people to Kimberley, many who have different ailments or issues to resolve. I tell everyone it is hard to describe the progress we have made because of vibrational healing; you really have to experience and feel it.

But hopefully I have managed to evidence in this the real clinical benefits we have experienced. Isobel is next scanned in August 2015 and when Kimberley writes her second book I am looking forward to writing another chapter where I will be able to formally confirm that Isobel is cancer-free.

And just one last note from me. Kimberley and her healing gave us hope where there was despair and light where there was darkness. We stand together as a family because of her role in our lives. Cancer throws everything on its head but we will come out of this with some positives too and vibrational healing, and Kimberley is one of the biggest parts of that.

Testimonial and thankfulness from Isobel Hodgkinson

I first met Kimberley on Sunday 9 December 2014. She met us at the gate holding two little grey furry dogs. We have two dogs at home ourselves and I couldn't wait to jump out the car and stroke them. Kimberley told me their names were Piccio and Tifo and that they were toy poodles.

I hugged and played with them whilst Mummy and Daddy chatted with Kimberley. We then all went into her treatment room and to my joy Piccio and Tifo came too.

Kimberley's treatment room felt safe to me and it was funny seeing Daddy have a treatment, and I remember Ruby, Ted and I giggling as Daddy got himself ready to have his treatment with Kimberley.

Nothing that Kimberley did was scary and I was looking forward to my turn. Well, it has been my turn for ten months. I have been seeing Kimberley two to three times a week. I love seeing Kimberley, her room makes me feel so safe and her bed is so warm and cosy. When Kimberley treats me I can feel what she is doing around my body and I hear the bowls that she plays on me, while I am asleep, and I know I am getting better.

Piccio and Tifo have also been such loyal companions to me, they seem to sense when I have been overwhelmed with chemotherapy and other medications. I have just sat and cuddled them. Piccio and I have a special bond, he often lies by my side and I get such comfort from our bond.

Kimberley is an angel to me, we all call her our Angel Healer.

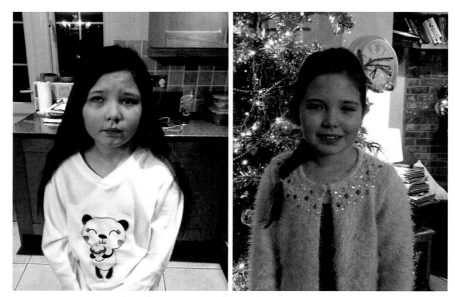

Isobel before (left) and after (right) treatment with Kimberley

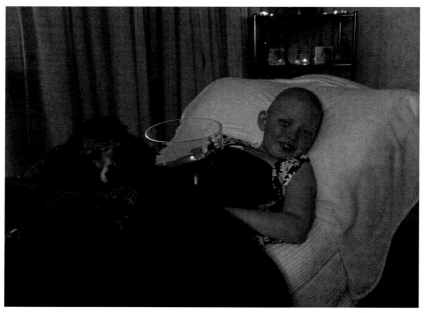

Isobel with Piccio during treatment

Update, October 2015, from Helen Hodgkinson

We received a letter from Isobel's consultant Kate Wheeler instructing us that Isobel would need a full body scan. The scan would show them how Isobel's cancer was doing and what the next lot of clinical protocol would be.

Isobel had her scan and as a family we were all very apprehensive on the results. Kimberley was reassuring us all that the scan would show that Isobel was cancer free. How do you know that, I asked? Kimberley answered: "I cannot feel it in her body any more." I must say Isobel looked very well. She had tons of energy and her body wasn't reacting like a body with cancer.

So on 1 October 2015 Ceri and I went to the follow up meeting to hear the results of the scan. We were both very apprehensive, as you can imagine, because Isobel was either clear of cancer or we were looking at another year of chemotherapy... Well, nothing prepared us for what we were about to hear. Kate, the consultant, said the scan showed that Isobel is in complete remission and cancer-free. This was confirmed by the full body MRI. Kate then confirmed that Isobel has been in full remission since early summer. She will be completing her maintenance programme (because it does what is says on the tin and will maintain her at her current state). Her all clear countdown has started early because of her progress with Kimberley's healing. It started at diagnosis on Nov 2014, rather then later, as would be the norm. So the final all-clear in the clinical sense should be in 2019. Kate has confirmed that she is 90% likely to get here.

Kimberley's healing has resulted in a number of extraordinary things:

1 *Early remission.*

2 *A more guaranteed all-clear.*

3 *Better able to cope with the clinical side of the treatment.*

4 *Healing the whole family allowed us all to deal with this hell much better.*

If you or your child is diagnosed with cancer, please, please contact Kimberley.*

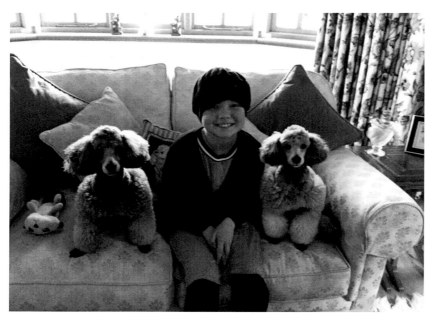

When Isobel got the results of the scan

* *Footnote from Kimberley:* The above outcome and the outcome of all the other testimonials have come about by these cancer patients putting my healing at the forefront of their protocol to becoming cancer free. Each patient has received an hour of my treatment four to seven times per week. This is the commitment required to maximize the chance of receiving an all-clear outcome.

Thankfulness from Isobel's dad, Ceri Hodgkinson

I was devastated when we were given the news that our first child Isobel was diagnosed with Ewing's (later re-diagnosed with non-Hodgkin's B cell lymphoma). As a Dad you would stand in front of a moving train to save the life of your children, as I sat there with the news sinking in, I felt the room swallowing me up and I was finding it hard to breathe.

Needing to be strong for Isobel and my wife Helen, I hid the fear that was taking over my senses. I could hear the exchange of voices but I must have zoned out. I came to, hearing Isobel asking if she could speak to someone of her own age that was going through the same treatment that she would be embarking on within days.

My daughter's consultant, Kate Wheeler, did put us in touch with another family whose young daughter had gone through chemotherapy. As it turned out my wife already knew the family so we made contact and agreed to meet the very next day. It was at this reunion that Joanne, the mother of the daughter that was under Kate Wheeler, suggested that it might be beneficial for us and Isobel to consider an alternative therapy route as well as the clinicians' route as she herself had taken her daughter to see Kimberley. My wife Helen jumped at the opportunity to take Kimberley's contact details and on arriving home we got in touch.

On 9 December 2014 we, as a family, all arrived at Kimberley's house. We were greeted with love and warmth, and immediately felt at ease in Kimberley's company. A plate of hot blueberry muffins were waiting for us, along with coffee and soft drinks for our children (we have three, Isobel, Ruby and Ted). After bringing Kimberley up to speed on Isobel's diagnosis, we followed Kimberley into her treatment room. Kimberley suggested that Isobel watched Mummy or Daddy having a treatment, so Isobel would know what to expect. There ensued a small discussion on who should have the treatment, and I was the winner. I am a builder by trade and definitely a man's man. I had never, until this moment, even considered anything alternative, but to my surprise I felt amazing afterwards but couldn't put into words how I felt. It felt like a lifting of all of the fear that was locked inside me. I reassured Isobel that she would love it.

I decided to take Ruby and Ted out of the room and left my wife with Isobel. Kimberley proceeded to give Isobel her first treatment. When Isobel came out an hour later with her mum, it was immediately obvious there was a change in both Isobel and her mum. They both seemed calmer, and more at peace. Isobel had not only been diagnosed with non-Hodgkin's B cell lymphoma, she also had a tumour growing in her eye socket which had completed distorted her face and was impinging on her eyesight. After her second session, three days later, the tumour on her eye socket was no longer visible and the swelling on her face had disappeared.

We all love going to Kimberley's. We feel so at peace in her company and in her treatment room; Isobel cannot wait to go there. Over the ten months that we have been under Kimberley's care, I have got to know her husband Joe very well, he is also a very kind and giving person as at any time he can have two families in and out of his home, and if Kimberley is tied up, Joe steps in and shows the same love and generosity that Kimberley does. I shudder to think where we would be, as a family, right now if Isobel hadn't had the fortitude to ask Kate is she could put us in touch with a family who had gone through the same nightmare that we were embarking on.

Isobel loves coming to see Kimberley and I firmly believe that it is the treatment she receives from her that has allowed Isobel's body to cope and heal so well. Isobel is still going to school and taking part in physical activities. Her medical team in Oxford are amazed at the progress she is making and as I write this she is now Isobel is entering into the maintenance phase of her clinical treatment.

As a final note I would encourage you all, if you are going through the brutal journey of cancer, please contact Kimberley immediately. Kimberley and Joe have done so much for my family; I know we will be great friends for life.

I am a true believer in we cross paths with people who are going to have an impact on our lives; but knowing it and trusting it are two very different things.

What you are about to read is a true account of paths crossing.

In 2008 I was diagnosed with an Anaplastic Oligastrocytoma, WHO grade 3 (Brain Tumour) at the age of 38. My life expectancy with treatment was two to five years. Fortunately I responded well to treatment and the disease remained stable for seven years.

I am a landscape gardener and as you can imagine I do meet a lot of people sporadically in my job, as well as fellow gardeners. One such fellow gardener was a lady called Bronwyn. Bronwyn was a lovely New Zealand lady, married with four children to a great guy called Carl. For as long as I have known Bronwyn she has always wanted to return to her native country of New Zealand. Well, in September of 2013, Bronwyn announced that she was going to return to New Zealand, with her family, and asked if I would be interested in taking over some of her gardens as she had become quite attached to a few of them, and she knew I would keep them well maintained.

One such garden happened to be that of a lady called Kimberley. Bronwyn mentioned that if I was to see a sign saying 'Treatment in progress' I would need to be as quiet as possible. Not being a curious man, I never really asked what Kimberley was doing, so a couple of months before Bronwyn was about to leave, my wife and I popped over with Bronwyn to Kimberley's and we were introduced.

Kimberley explained that she helped heal cancer patients and I flippantly said, "Gosh if only I knew you in 2008 when I was diagnosed with a brain tumour." Breaking the ice at that moment, we all laughed. I explained that in 2008 my brain tumour was removed and since then I was healthy and living a full and happy life. Kimberley said that if ever I felt off-colour and I wanted to try a treatment or two with her, just to ask. A few weeks later we bid Bronwyn and her family farewell and I started attending Kimberley's garden.

Within months of me taking over Kimberley's garden, I was aware that I wasn't quite up to par and I was struggling to hear, and being a man I let it slide for a while until January 2015 when I was sent a letter for a routine check-up scan. To my horror the scan showed that my tumour had begun to grow again and had infiltrated my ear canal and the frontal lobe of my brain.

The plan of action from my clinicians was to wait for a surgery date. As my wife Sally and I left the hospital and drove home, the conversation was all about how long the wait for a surgery date would be, would I survive? And would Kimberley's treatment make any difference? We both agreed that we had nothing to lose by popping over and asking Kimberley for her help.

When we arrived at Kimberley's front door she greeted us with friendship and love. She was a little puzzled, however, as it was winter time and she wasn't expecting me for another three months. We were warmly ushered into her kitchen for a cup of tea and a piece of cake. Being a man, I felt a bit awkward at first as we don't often like to ask for *help, so my wife Sally did all the talking. As the severity of the reason we were there hit Kimberley, her eyes filled up with tears and she said she would do whatever it took to help me back on the road to recovery and said, "Let's start treatment now".*

Kimberley suggested that I have three one-hourly sessions a week with her and she would continue this pattern of treatment right to the very end of whatever my clinicians suggested, even if it involved chemotherapy and radiation.

So I started my weekly sessions with Kimberley and I began to feel on top of the world. My deafness started to subside, as did my other symptoms. My hearing returned fully after a period of treatment. Our home life was getting back to normality and life was good. Towards the end of March I received a letter from Southampton Hospital to say I needed a scan to prep me for surgery which was going to take place the following week. Feeling on top of the world this news did not overly concern me as I knew I had three more treatments with Kimberley before my surgery.

I had my scan and we waited to see my consultant. As we were called into his room Sally and I noticed he had an air of surprise about him. He asked how I was feeling and I said, "I feel great."

"Well," he said, "You may feel even better after you see the dramatic changes from the scan we took of you in January to the scan you have just had this morning."

Sally and I glanced at each other and gave a knowing nod as we knew Kimberley's treatment was doing something extraordinary. The scan showed a miraculous change. It showed that the tumour had changed in shape and was being pulled away from the brain into the cavity that was there from previous surgery seven years earlier. The surgeon was so pleased with the scan results that he was confident of an easier resection than the last operation in 2008. I had surgery at the end of March 2015.

I was only in hospital for three days, post-surgery, and then I was allowed to come home. I left hospital barely able to walk and could only mobilise very short distances with the aid of a Zimmer frame. Sally and I knew that I needed to get myself back into Kimberley's treatment room as I knew she would reverse the paralysis that I was left with after surgery. On resuming my treatment with Kimberley I was able to walk with a walking stick and people would comment that I was radiating good health and mobility. My surgical wound healed beautifully and I had none of the infection issues I had after my previous surgery in 2008. My clinicians suggested I start a small treatment of chemotherapy which Kimberley's treatment supported me through and I have been having, to date, two to three treatments a week which I am very grateful for and to be honest I never miss them.

I had, on 7 September 2015, a follow-up scan, which shows there are microscopic malignant cells in the brain. Kimberley is continuing to see me. I cannot say or prove that Kimberley's treatment will cure cancer but I cannot say or prove that it will not either. What I can say is that I radiated health and great wellbeing whilst undergoing the horrors of chemotherapy.

I have had outstanding medical and nursing care throughout my treatment which has ultimately kept me alive and well and which both Sally and I are eternally grateful for. However, I truly believe that Kimberley has given me something far greater and it is hard to describe.

My wife Sally, who is a Junior Sister of a busy acute surgical ward at Basingstoke Hospital, a full-time mum to our active and energetic four-year-old daughter as well as my full-time carer, often pops along with me whilst I have my treatment and just by Sally being in the room with me, soaking up Kimberley's healing energy, she has benefited as well. Our friends and family often comment that Sally should be on her knees with the stress of it all, but she is not. Sally puts it down to her visits to Kimberley.

Kimberley has suggested I continue with my healing sessions with her for the foreseeable future. I am happy to tell you that I will be resuming my full-time gardening business next spring and I am looking forward to a long healthy and prosperous life.

Sally and I feel extremely blessed that our paths have crossed with Kimberley's and she will forever stay in our hearts as a very dear friend. Throughout our journey Sally was the only one working full-time when she could. Kimberley has never burdened us with the worry of her fees. She has treated me, and is happy to continue treating me, free of charge. Kimberley is one of the warmest, loving and most caring people I know.

She is very enthusiastic about her model of healing and how it can benefit cancer patients, and Sally and I champion her approach to the most devastating journey you may have to undertake in your life.

Thank you Kimberley.

Sally's thankfulness

When we found out Steve's cancer had reappeared in his brain, I was surprised as he had been doing so well for so long. I knew I would be his rock despite my busy schedule as a Junior Sister on the acute surgical ward at my local hospital. I have always been a champion of holistic therapy and when we were introduced to Kimberley I definitely encouraged Steve to take up Kimberley's offer of help. I do believe the months of treatment he has received from Kimberley has helped enormously and even though I cannot say Kimberley's treatment cured Steve's cancer, I cannot say or prove that it hasn't either. I do wish more oncologists would embrace Kimberley's kind of alternative therapy as I feel it has its place alongside the clinical root. I do like to pop in on Steve's treatment when I get a chance as I know the healing I receive helps me cope with the stresses and strains of my job and my role as a full time mum to my four-year-old daughter. We as a family are very grateful to Kimberley for all she has done, and is still doing, to this day and beyond.

Also Available

Kimberley's healing and chill out CDs and her healing oils are available through her website: www.healingbykimberley.com

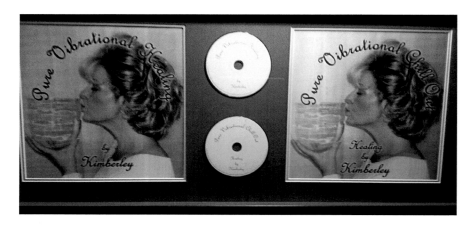

Kimberley's 'Healing' CD has been created to help the body and mind to become calmer. It can aid in a good night's sleep and calms and settles newborns in their new surroundings at home. It is also excellent for our four legged family members.

Kimberley's 'Chill Out' CD has been created to be listened to while in the car and in the home. It reduces stress and will give your whole body a sense of calm and well-being.

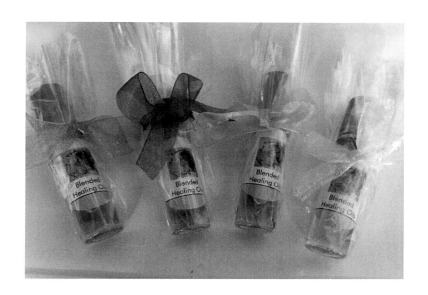

Kimberley has also created her own blend of healing and relaxing oils. These oils have been created and blended by Kimberley. Each bottle contains over 18 different essentials oils to enable adults and children alike, to sleep well and keep you calm throughout the day.

Suggested Reading

If you have enjoyed thinking out of the box, then here are some suggestions for extra reading:

- *THE HEALING POWER OF SOUND* by Mitchell L. Gaynor M.D.

- *THE COMPLETE IDIOT'S GUIDE TO THE AKASHIC RECORD* by Dr Synthia Andrews, ND and Colin Andrews

- *BAD PHARMA* by Ben Goldacre

- *BAD SCIENCE* by Ben Goldacre

- *CANCER IS NOT A DISEASE – IT'S A SURVIVAL MECHANISM* by Andreas Moritz

- *YOU ARE THE PLACEBO* by Dr Joe Dispenza

- *EAT RIGHT FOR YOUR BLOOD TYPE* by Dr Peter J. D'Adamo with Catherine Whitney

- *ANATOMY OF THE SPIRIT* by Caroline Myss, PhD

- *THE POWER OF NOW* by Eckhart Tolle